Criminal Poisoning

FORENSIC ◊ SCIENCE ◊ AND ◊ MEDICINE

Steven B. Karch, MD, SERIES EDITOR

Criminal Poisoning: *Investigational Guide for Law Enforcement, Toxicologists, Forensic Scientists, and Attorneys,* by *JOHN H. TRESTRAIL III,* 2000

A Physician's Guide to Clinical Forensic Medicine, edited by *MARGARET M. STARK,* 2000

Toxicology of Herbal Products, edited by *MELANIE JOHNS CUPP,* 2000

Brain Imaging in Substance Abuse: *Research, Clinical, and Forensic Applications* edited by *MARC J. KAUFMAN,* 2000

CRIMINAL POISONING

INVESTIGATIONAL GUIDE FOR LAW ENFORCEMENT, TOXICOLOGISTS, FORENSIC SCIENTISTS, AND ATTORNEYS

JOHN HARRIS TRESTRAIL, III, RPH, FAACT, DABAT

REGIONAL POISON CENTER, GRAND RAPIDS, MI

999 Riverview Drive, Suite 208
Totowa, New Jersey 07512

For additional copies, pricing for bulk purchases, and/or information about other Humana titles, contact Humana at the above address or at any of the following numbers: Tel.: 973-256-1699; Fax: 973-256-8341; E-mail: humana@humanapr.com, or visit our Website: http://humanapress.com

Cover design by Patricia F. Cleary

This publication is printed on acid-free paper. ∞
ANSI Z39.48-1984 (American National Standards Institute) Permanence of Paper for Printed Library Materials).

Printed in the United States of America. 10 9 8 7 6 5 4 3 2 1

Library of Congress Cataloging-in-Publication Data

Trestrail, John H.
Criminal poisoning: investigational guide for law enforcement, toxicologists, forensic scientists, and attorneys/John H. Trestrail, III.
p. cm.—(Forensic science; 2)
Includes bibliographical references and index.
ISBN 0-89603-592-1 (alk. paper)
1. Forensic toxicology. 2. Poisoning. I. Title. II. Series.
RA1228.T74 2000
615.9—dc21 99-35530
CIP

Preface

Passion [poison] often makes fools of clever men; sometimes even makes clever men of fools.—***La Rochefoucauld***

This book represents a pioneering work dealing exclusively with poisons in the hands of the murderer, tamperer, and terrorist.

One of the oldest offensive killing weapons developed by humanity, after the stick, stone, and fist, were the poisons. Yet, after nearly 5000 years of recorded history, no in-depth work has ever been produced dealing exclusively with poisons as weapons for homicide. The author's review of the international literature has revealed only a few scattered scientific papers dealing with the psychology of the poisoner, and books on medical jurisprudence and forensic investigation have devoted only a few pages to this important subject, usually stating that it is a "rare" occurrence. How do we know the true rarity of the use of poisons for homicide? All one has to do is look at the number of poisonings that are first documented only after the exhumation of the deceased to raise the logical question: If we missed this one, how many more have been missed? If all those buried in our cemeteries who had been poisoned could raise their hands, we would probably be aghast at the numbers!

For years, the homicidal poisoner has remained shrouded in mystery. What little we think we know about the criminal poisoner represents only the tip of an iceberg, with the majority of our knowledge still remaining hidden under the surface. My hope is that this work will serve as a valuable tool in the hands of the criminal investigator, forensic scientist, toxicologist, and attorney, and better increase our chances of avenging each victim of a homicidal poisoner.

Unfortunately, a copy of this work is eventually bound to wind up in the hands of a potential criminal poisoner, and the individual may gain some information to use in planning and attempting to escape the crime. But the trade off is that law enforcement at the same time will now have in this work detailed information that should prove of assistance in dealing more effectively with this almost invisible crime.

Homicide by poisoning is one of the most difficult types of cases for the death investigator and medical expert to prove. It has been stated that poisonings are rarely encountered, accounting for only 3–6% of homicides. However, I believe that these homicides do not rarely occur, but rather are rarely detected.

The main problem is that in poisonings, the investigator often has no visible signs of trauma to indicate that the death is other than natural. Bullets leave holes, knives leave cuts, and clubs leave bruises, but the poisoner covers the murder with a blanket of invisibility. Important clues are usually buried with the victim. Because poisons are offensive weapons, not defensive weapons, often the crime scene may seem nonexistent.

As the French scientist Louis Pasteur once said, "Chance favors the prepared mind." In this spirit, it is hoped that the contents of this work will so prepare the mind of all criminal investigators, and therefore greatly increase their chances of solving this type of crime.

For as the poem on p. viii tries to tell, we each must become a "Toxic Avenger," and bring to justice those individuals who have chosen this most secretive mode of homicide. It makes no difference whether a victim was killed with a knife, a gun, a bomb, or a poison; each and every one deserves the fullest justice our society can deliver!

John Harris Trestrail, III, RPh, FAACT, DABAT

DISCLAIMER

This publication is intended to serve the reader with general background information representing various aspects of toxicology as it applies to modern litigation. However, this is not intended to serve as a substitute for intensive research respecting various issues as each case must be approached on a case-by-case basis. Some cases will require intensive research independent of this work.

The author would like to humbly dedicate
this first ever work to his parents,
***John Harris** and **Edith (McClay) Trestrail**,*
for emigrating from England and Ireland to America,
which provided unlimited professional opportunities
for their two children, and who through their continued
support and educational encouragement over the years
allowed their children to grow and contribute
in the vocations they chose to follow.

Also, this work is dedicated to the author's wife
***Mary,** and his children, **John** and **Amanda**,*
who allowed him to passionately follow his love
for the subject of toxicology, even though at many times
they must have considered it somewhat
eccentric and bizarre.

ACKNOWLEDGMENTS

The author would like formally to acknowledge and thank the following individuals and groups who were of great assistance in the research and preparation of this manuscript: Mr. Arthur E. Westveer, Instructor at the FBI Academy, for his encouragement and taking the author under his tutelage to teach him the fundamentals of death investigation, gained through his many years as a Detective Lieutenant in the Homicide Unit of the Baltimore City Police Department; the dedicated members of the Behavioral Sciences Unit at the FBI Academy, in Quantico, VA, for their continued dialog, excellent learning opportunities, and technical support; toxicologist Dr. Bernard H. Eisenga, PHD, MD, for reading the various drafts of this manuscript and offering his constructive comments; and the staff of the Spectrum Health Regional Poison Center and its host hospital, Spectrum Health, in Grand Rapids, MI for their encouragement in allowing the author to follow his passion to carry out his monumental forensic project.

The Toxic Avenger

by

John Harris Trestrail, III, RPh, FAACT, DABAT
Toxicologist

From the grave, if lips could speak
the person who was, pleads—you must seek
the individual who had my trust,
and thru deceit and cunning into the grave did thrust
this body once alive and well,
now silenced by death, who cannot tell
my death was NOT what all thought then,
for a poison brought my life to end!

Avenge me now, for you alone
can find the truth beneath this stone.
Look close and the clues you will see
that tell the tale of what killed me.
For you must tell all others now,
That this was MURDER—and tell them how!
For if no one looks to find what's here,
an injustice was done to a life so dear.
If now only you could hear,
my muted pleadings to make wants clear.
I'd speak as plain as it could be.
Since I can't—You must AVENGE ME!

Contents

List of Tables

Chapter 1

Poisoners Throughout History

> *"I maintain that though you would often in the fifteenth century have heard the snobbish Roman say, in a would-be off-hand tone, 'I am dining with the Borgias tonight', no Roman was ever able to say, 'I dined last night with the Borgias.'"* —*And Even Now,* Max Beerbohm

It is safe to say that poisoners have always been part of society, continue to be with us now, and will likely be with us in the future. To better understand these offenders, it is important for us to understand how our knowledge of poisons has developed and has been passed down throughout history, in the various cultures and societies of the world.

1.1. POISONS IN ANCIENT TIMES

1.1.1. Introduction

The first homicidal poisoner is now clearly lost in the mists of time, but one can certainly speculate on the type of person and incident that led to the possession of this knowledge. Certainly he or she was a member of an early tribe of ancient humanity who first noticed the negative effects that exposure to certain substances had on living organisms. Perhaps it began with the observation that, shortly after consuming a plant, fungus, or mineral, an animal or fellow tribal member became ill and possibly died. This reasoning individual was able to conclude cause and effect by the method "*post hoc ergo propter hoc*" ("after this, therefore on account of this"); this method is usually considered an illogical form of reasoning, but here is quite correctly applied. This observation allowed the proper determination of the potential for the deleterious effects that would result from exposure to a certain substance originating from an animal, vegetable, or mineral source. Any individual who obtained this knowledge of poison effects would certainly possess a great power among fellow tribal members. Perhaps the knowledge could have been used for the good of the group, as with the development of poisons for hunting, but the knowledge could certainly have been as easily used for homicidal purposes. This knowledge of poisons led eventually to power, the power to mystery, and the mystery to the fear of those individuals holding the ability to kill with such an invisible weapon. It is probable that this powerful knowledge was kept secret among a very select group of shamanistic individuals. Whomever this individual was, the knowledge he possessed was passed among selected members of the inner power circle, by word-of-mouth, down through countless generations.

Let us travel backward in time to look at various ancient peoples and their knowledge of poisons, and especially the use of these substances for the purpose of homicide.

1.1.2. The Sumerians

Our first stop to the past is with the Sumerians, peoples living in Mesopotamia (modern day Iraq) around 2500 BCE. It is well known that there has been a knowledge and interest in the subject of poisons as far back as their early recorded history. Decipherings of the Sumerians' ancient cuneiform clay documents have revealed that they worshiped a deity of noxious poisons known to them as "Gula." She was the first known, recorded spirit associated with poisons.

1.1.3. The Ancient Egyptians

As early as 3000 BCE, the Egyptian King Menes studied the properties of poisonous plants (Smith, 1952). An ancient Egyptian papyrus recorded the incantation, "repeat not the name I.A.O., under the penalty of the peach." The Egyptians may have known that the seed kernel of the peach, and other members of the botanical genus Prunus (including the cherry, apricot, and bitter almond), contain plant compounds known today as "cyanogenic glycosides," which can release toxic cyanide compounds in the presence of water and the proper plant enzyme. The Egyptians even believed that their gods were susceptible to the effects of poisonous entities. They believed that their god "Ra" nearly succumbed from the effects of a venomous snakebite, and that "Horus" suffered a fatal outcome from the sting of a scorpion. In 525 BCE, Psammentius, the King of Egypt, was forced to drink the then-believed poisonous substance "bull's blood," which allegedly caused his immediate death. Zopyrus, a physician in Alexandria, concocted a general poison antidote that consisted of 30–50 various ingredients.

1.1.4. The Hebrews

Some scholars believe that the witches mentioned in the Old Testament were sorcerers and poison vendors. The Hebrews even had words for some of our dangerous poisons: "*Sam*" (Arsenic), "*Boschka*" (Aconite), and "*Son*" (Ergot). Although the use of poisoned arrows is mentioned in the Bible (in the book of Job) there are no references in the Old or New Testaments to the homicidal use of poisons (Bombaugh, 1899).

1.1.5. The Asian Indians

In the earliest writings from ancient India, one can begin to see discussions of the incidence of homicidal poisoning and its investigation. Two of the earliest writings on the subject of poisons, dating from 600–100 BCE, were the *Charaka Sambita* and the *Susruta Sambita*. Another document, The Veda, gives the physician specific directions in the detection of poisoners:

> *"He does not answer questions, or the answers are evasive. He speaks nonsense, rubs the great toe along the ground and shivers. His face is discolored. He rubs the roots of the hair with his fingers and he tries by every means to leave the house. The food which is suspected should be given to animals. It is necessary for the practitioner to have knowledge of the symptoms of the different poisons and their antidotes, as the enemies of the Raja, bad women and ungrateful servants sometimes mix poison with food."*

It has even been speculated by some scholars that the Indian practice of "*suttee,*" in which the living widow was burned along with the corpse of her late husband, might have had some basis in attempting to discourage conjugal homicide (Meek, 1928).

1.1.6. Nicander of Colophon

Nicander (204–135 BCE), a physician, compiled the first poison pharmacopeia while serving as personal attendant to Attalus III, the King of Pergamum (in modern Turkey). His favorite antidote consisted of viper parts seasoned with aromatic herbs and fruits (consisting mostly of ginger, cinnamon, myrrh, iris, and gentian). This antidote probably has no toxicological basis for its effectiveness by today's standards. He also wrote two poems on poisons: the "*Theriaca,*" consisting of 1000 lines dealing with poisonous animals, and the "*Alexipharmaca,*" consisting of 600 lines dealing with the subject of antidotes.

1.1.7. Philon of Tarsus

Philon was a physician who developed one of the most long-lived antidotal potions for poisoning, which was called the "*Philonium Romanorum.*" This antidotal concoction consisted of multiple herbs (Spikenard, Henbane, Pyrethrum, Euphorbia, and Saffron). Once again, it had no toxicological basis for its effectiveness by today's standards.

1.1.8. Mithridates

Mithridates, King of Pontus (in modern Turkey), lived around 100 BCE and had the reputation of knowing more about poisons and their proper antidotes than any other person of his time. He was very concerned with the possibility of his assassination by poison, and experimented with poisons and antidotes on himself as well as captured prisoners. He developed a so-called "universal" antidote, which was called "*Mithridatum*" in his honor. This antidote remained so popular in the minds of the people that it was still available in Italian pharmacies up through the 17th century. Once again, looking at the ingredients of this mixture with today's toxicological knowledge, it is obvious that little protection could be obtained from Mithridates' antidote.

1.1.9. The Greeks

The Greeks gave us the word "toxicon,"— used to denote poison, —from their word signifying a bow, which in warfare was used to shoot poisoned arrows at the enemy. From this Greek word comes all of the words in use today to denote poison: "toxicology," "toxic," "intoxicated," and so on. If one were to talk to an ancient Greek who admitted to being intoxicated, it would not have the same meaning that the word has today, because he would be describing a physical condition resulting from being poisoned by an arrow.

Medea, a sorceress and the priestess of Hecate in Greek mythology; was credited as the first to the use the plant known as "Meadow Saffron" (*Colchicum autumnale L.*) as a poison. Today, we know this plant contains the very potent poison Colchicine, used in modern medicine as a remedy for gout. In the classic literary work of the Greek, Homer's *Odyssey*, one finds a discussion of one of the first great sorceresses, Circe, who used poisons and potions to subdue men to her ways.

The most famous of the Greek poisoners was Olympias, the wife of Philip of Macedon and the mother of Alexander the Great. She was involved in the deaths of Aridaeus, his wife Eurydice, Nicanor, and many other prominent men of Macedonia.

The Greeks also developed what was known as the "Athenian State Poison," concocted from the very poisonous plant more commonly known today as "Poison Hemlock" (*Conium maculatum* L.). This very toxic plant containing the poison "Coniine," was reportedly used to execute the philosopher Socrates for his crime of corrupting the youth of Athens with his philosophical teachings.

Aristotle, in his writings of the period, described the preparation and use of arrow poisons by the Scythians, in which they allowed the bodies of snakes to decay and combined the exuding liquid with the clear fluid from decomposing blood. This mixture was then applied to arrows for use in battles. The greatest danger from this material was likely owing to septicemia (blood poisoning) from bacterial invasion.

It is interesting to note that a review of the writings of the famous Greek physician Hippocrates reveals no information on criminal poisoning. He did, however, make his students swear that they would not traffic in poisons in their practice of the medical arts.

During the Greek period, the Court of Areopagus was assigned the function of dealing with trials for poisoning cases.

The physician Galen (131–201 AD) compounded an antidote called "Nut Theriac," which was to be used as a remedy for bites, stings, and other poisons. This antidote consisted of plant parts and salt, mixed into a porridge.

1.1.10. The Romans

The ancient Romans documented the grand scale use of poisons, on a grand scale, for homicidal purposes. As early as 331 BCE, according to the writer Livy, there was an outbreak of homicidal poisoning in high circles of Roman society. One of the most infamous poisoners of the time was a woman named Locusta, who was the personal poisoner of Emperor Nero. With her assistance and advice, Nero murdered his brother Britanicus with cyanide containing natural compounds, and also murdered his mother and several wives. Livia, who was the wife of Emperor Augustus, used the Belladonna plant as a homicidal weapon. Agrippina, the wife of Claudius, killed him by injecting poisons into figs he then ate. Eventually 170 Roman women were convicted and punished for their homicidal poisoning activities.

So prevalent was the use of the "Wolfsbane" plant (*Aconitum napellus L.)*, with its very toxic alkaloid aconitine, that the Emperor Trajan (98–117 AD) eventually banned the growth of this plant in Roman domestic gardens. In fact, the writer Ovid refered to aconite as the "step-mother's poison."

In 82 BCE, the ruler Sulla issued an edict known as the "Lex Cornelia" against assassination by poison. This edict was the first legislative enactment in history against the use of poison as a means of homicide.

1.1.11. The "Italian School of Poisoners"

Deep within the psyche of the Italians of the Middle Ages existed the knowledge and will to use poisons to obtain wealth and power. In the year 1419, members of a group known as the Venetian "Council of Ten" carried out murder by poison for a fee. Three of their recipes for poison weapons are preserved as the "secreta secretissima," in archives dating from 1540–1544 AD. Chief ingredients included corrosive sublimate (mercuric chloride), white arsenic (arsenic trioxide), arsenic trisulfide, and arsenic trichloride. In Venice and Rome, in the 15th to 17th centuries, there were schools for students who wished to become poisoners.

The name Borgia is the first that comes to mind with this location and period of time. The leader of this poisoning clan was one Rodrigo Borgia, born in 1431, who went on to become Pope Alexander VI. Among his five children were Cesare and Lucrezia, who most people associate with murder-by-poison plots. In fact, Lucrezia, who died at the age of 39, probably never killed anyone. However, her brother Cesare, who died at the age of 32, was responsible for dozens of murders that used poison as the instrument. The poison most frequently used by the Borgias was arsenic, which they used in the form of a poison they called "La Cantrella," a mixture of arsenic and phosphorus. It is believed that their weapon was prepared as follows:

> *"A hog was killed with arsenic. Its abdomen was opened and sprinkled with more of the same drug. The animal was then allowed to putrefy. The liquor which trickled from the decaying carcass was collected and evaporated to a powder" (Meek, 1928).*

With the secret popularity of a piece of jewelry known as a poison ring, certainly no one aware of the Borgia's knowledge of poisons would want to take dinner with them without some consternation about the possible consequences.

Around 1650 another famous Italian poisoner of the era, Madame Giulia Toffana, produced and sold a mixture to would-be users called "Aqua Toffana," thought to have been a solution of arsenic trioxide. She was credited with over 600 successful poisonings, and admitted to being involved in the poisoning of two Popes, Pius III and Clement IV.

In 1659, the poisoner Hieronyma Spara formed a society in which she taught women how to murder their husbands by means of poisons. She dispensed her poison in small vials labeled "Manna of St. Nicholas of Bari."

Catherine de Medici, who became the bride of the French King Henry II, was credited with carrying the Italian knowledge about poisons outside of the country. In fact, the King was so afraid of her poisoning powers and abilities that a "unicorn's horn" (most likely the tusk of a marine mammal called the Narwal) then thought to be an antidote again poisons, became part of the official regal dowry. It was Catherine who introduced the proven Italian methods of poisoning into France by means of her accomplices, the Florentines Rene Bianco and Cosme Ruggieri. Catherine is usually credited as being involved with the homicidal poisonings of Jeanne d'Albret, Queen of Navarre; the Cardinal of Lorraine; Coffe, a Marshal of France; and the Duc d'Anjou.

1.1.12. The "French School of Poisoners"

The most notorious maker of poisons in the 17th century was a man named Antonio Exili (a.k.a. Eggidi). During his imprisonment in the Bastille, he taught his skills to a fellow prisoner named Gaudin de Sainte-Croix. Upon release from prison, Sainte-Croix teamed up with a very greedy woman by the name of Marie Madeleine, the Marchioness de Brinvilliers. They soon experimented with many poisonous compounds, such as arsenic, sugar of lead, corrosive sublimate, tartar emetic, and copper sulfate. In fact, the Marchioness even took their formulations into the hospitals of the time, mixed in gifts of food and drink for the sick, in order to study the effectiveness of their poisonous weapons. To gain property and wealth, she allegedly murdered her father, two brothers, and a sister. Found guilty of these crimes, she was executed in Paris in 1676.

Another of the French poisoners was Catherine Deshayes (a.k.a. La Voisin), who was an abortionist, and considered a sorceress of the time. She provided poisons to women so that they could do away with their spouses. One of her popular poisons was known as "La Poudre de Succession" ("Inheritance Powder"). This poison was thought to have had a base of arsenic, mixed with aconite, belladonna, and opium. She was probably one of the last poisoners for hire. Deshayes accepted a sizeable commission to poison Louis XIV, but—having been unsuccessful—was found guilty of the attempt on the King's life. Her punishment, after severe torture, was to be burned at the stake.

An investigative organization known as the "Chambre Ardente" ("The Fiery Room"), operating in France (1679–1682) under the reign of Louis XIV, was formed to deal with criminal poisoners. During the Chambre's operation, it investigated 442 persons and ordered 367 arrests. Of those individuals investigated, 36 were executed, 23 banished, and 218 imprisoned. It was, in effect, a poisoner's "Inquisition."

Through the ages, many other poisoners operated around the world, in various countries.

- In 1596, Edward Squires was hired by Spain to poison Queen Elizabeth I by smearing an opium-based poison on the pommel of her saddle.

- In 1613, the Countess of Somerset was found guilty for utilizing "Corrosive Sublimate" (mercuric chloride) in a mass conspiracy to murder Sir Thomas Overbury while he was imprisoned in the Tower of London.
- In 1776, Thomas Hickey attempted to assassinate George Washington by poisoning a dish of green peas. Foiled in his attempt, he was hanged, becoming the first American executed for treason.

1.2. POISONERS IN THE MODERN ERA

We should not fool ourselves into thinking that poisoners operated only in the past, because they have continued their nefarious crimes into the present day. What follows are brief vignettes of some infamous poisoners that have, fortunately, been caught in their evil deeds, and we can learn a great deal from their cases. These cases, arranged in chronological order, have been selected by the author from his collection of incidents of homicidal poisonings as revealing various important facets of this type of crime.

1.2.1. William Palmer, MD, "The Rugeley Poisoner" (1855)

In 1855, Dr. William Palmer, of Rugeley, Staffordshire was a physician with a gambling problem. Motivated by the gain of easy money, he poisoned fellow horseracing gambler named John Parsons Cook. Palmer's poison of choice was the heavy metallic element antimony. Ultimately uncovered in his crime, he was put on trial. Interestingly enough, the trial had to be moved from the small town of Rugeley to London, because the change in venue was deemed necessary in order to obtain a more fair trial. (The legislative action for this move is still called the "Palmer Act" in England.) Dr. Palmer was convicted, and it is very possible that he was involved with as many as 14 others murders. He was hanged for his crime on June 14, 1856.

1.2.2. Edward William Pritchard, MD, "The Philandering Poisoner" (1865)

Glasgow, Scotland, in 1865, found this physician with a mistress. To eliminate his wife Mary Jane Palmer, he poisoned her and her mother, Mrs. Taylor, by using antimony in the form of the compound "Tartar Emetic." As the attending physician, he then conveniently certified the deaths of both women as resulting from gastrointestinal disturbances. An anonymous letter sent to the authorities eventually led to the arrest of Dr. Pritchard, and having being found guilty of the crimes, he was hanged on July 28, 1865, the last public hanging in Scotland.

1.2.3. George Henry Lamson, MD, "The Slight-of-Hand Poisoner" (1881)

Dr. George Henry Lamson was an English physician who suffered from an addiction to morphine and was in need of funds. In order to bring family estate funds into his domestic control, in December 1881, he selected as his victim his 18-year-old handicapped brother-in-law, Percy Malcolm John. While visiting John, and having tea and a Dundee raisin cake, he made a big deal of showing his relative a new American invention, the gelatin capsule, stating that it would make taking medicine much easier. To illustrate his point, he filled a capsule with sugar, and asked John to take it. A few hours later, after Dr. Lamson left by train for London, John began to suffer from severe stomach distress, and soon died. Dr. Lamson was eventually caught and charged, after trying to bribe the newspapers with inside knowledge of John's death. How did the poison get into the victim? Not in the capsule; Dr. Lamson had carefully tampered with some of the raisins in the slice of Dundee cake given to John, using the powerful alkaloidal poison aconite. His reward for this crime was his hanging on April 28, 1882.

1.2.4. Thomas Neill Cream, MD, "The Lambeth Poisoner" (1891)

The case of Dr. Thomas Neill Cream presents us with a rather unique motive. Dr. Cream was a sadist and moral degenerate, who took out his perverse feelings on prostitutes in the Lambeth area of London. His *modus operandi* was to offer capsules containing strychnine to the unfortunate victims under the guise that it was a medication to improve their complexions. The victims quickly died agonizing deaths. London, in its post-Jack-the-Ripper climate, soon named this unknown and demented serial killer the "Lambeth Poisoner." Cream eventually drew attention to himself when he offered to reveal to the authorities the identity of the infamous Lambeth Poisoner for a sum of many thousands of pounds. Placed on trial, it took the jury only 12 minutes to return a guilty verdict, and Cream was hanged on November 15, 1892.

1.2.5. Cordelia Botkin, "The Scorned Poisoner" (1898)

A "femme-fatale," Cordelia Botkin chose to poison her feminine rival, the wife of her paramour. In San Francisco, California, Cordelia had begun a romantic relationship with John Dunning, a war correspondent for the Associated Press. In 1898, John was assigned to cover the breaking war in Cuba, and informed his mistress that he would not be returning to her, but to his wife (the daughter of a state Senator) and family in Dover, Delaware. On August 9, 1898, an unsolicited box of chocolate candies arrived at the Dunning home in Delaware, addressed to Mrs. Dunning. Mary Dunning shared the crudely formed candies with her sister Mrs. Joshua Deane, and Mrs. Deane's two children. Shortly thereafter, all four people became violently ill, and subsequently the two older women succumbed from severe stomach ailments. With so many people becoming ill at the same time, the candies became suspect, and the remaining candy, as well as the victims, were found to be loaded with arsenic. John Dunning returned from Cuba, and he identified the handwriting on the package as Cordelia Botkin's; she was quickly arrested in California. After a jurisdictional fight between the states of California and Delaware, the trial was held in California, the location of the poisoner. Cordelia was found guilty of the crime and sentenced to life imprisonment, where she eventually died in San Quentin prison in 1909.

1.2.6. Johann Otto Hoch, "The Stockyards Bluebeard" (1892–1905)

Johann Otto Hoch was a serial killer who used arsenic as his weapon of choice. Hoch was an opportunist. Between 1892 and 1905, in various US states, he is thought to have murdered possibly 12 of his 24 wives, in order to obtain control of their financial assets. Hoch moved from town to town gaining the affections of new widows, endearing himself, and soon after marriage, taking control of their finances. The wife would then soon become ill, suffering from tremendous gastrointestinal upsets. After the wife's death, Johann would leave town with all the assets of the deceased. He would then move to a new town, check the obituaries in the local newspaper, select a new target, and begin the process again. Eventually, authorities were alerted to the similarities of the deaths. Hoch was arrested, whereupon it was found that he carried in his pocket a hollow fountain pen containing a white powder, which proved to be arsenic. He claimed that the poison was his exit dose to be used when he intended to commit suicide; however, upon further interrogation, he confessed to the many murders. Hoch stated "Marriage was purely a business proposition to me. When I found they had money, I went after that." He was found guilty of homicidal poisoning, and was hanged on February 23, 1906 in Chicago, Illinois.

1.2.7. Hawley Harvey Crippen, MD, "The Mild Mannered Murderer" (1910)

The Crippen case is one that contains many unusual aspects, and a few unanswered questions. Dr. Crippen, born in Coldwater, Michigan, in 1862, eventually went on to represent the firm "Munyon's Homeopathic Remedies," in London.

Dr. Crippen was a relatively small man, standing only 63 inches tall, and very quiet in demeanor. His second wife, Kunigunde Muckamotzki (a.k.a. Cora Turner, a.k.a. Belle Elmore), on the other hand,was a rather loud and brassy woman, with a very domineering personality. For several years prior to the disappearance of his wife, Dr. Crippen had been carrying on an affair with his office secretary, Ethel Le Neve. Sometime after the evening of January 31, 1910, Cora simply vanished. Things might have gone better for him if his mistress Ethel had not quickly moved into the Crippen home, and begun to wear Crippen's wife's clothes and jewelry. Soon, social acquaintances of the Crippens became suspicious and took their concerns to Scotland Yard. Upon questioning, Dr. Crippen changed his stories of his wife's whereabouts numerous times, claiming eventually that she had left him for another man, returned to America, and died. He might have gotten away with the crime if he hadn't panicked after being interrogated, and made a dash for Canada by ship. Ethel traveled with Crippen disguised as his young son, as she had cut her hair and was dressed in a young man's suit of clothes. Upon returning to the empty Crippen home, Inspector Dew of Scotland Yard serendipitously came upon a small piece of human tissue wrapped in a man's pajamas, buried under the floor of the coal cellar.

An international alarm quickly went out all across Europe for Crippen and Le Neve. On board ship, Dr. Crippen and Le Neve were soon identified by the ship's Captain, and a radio message was sent back to England of the presence of the fugitives among the passengers. This was the first time in history that the newly developed radio wireless was used in the apprehension of a criminal. Inspector Dew boarded a faster ship, and was waiting for the fugitive pair as they were ready to disembark in Canada. They were arrested and taken back to England to stand trial for the murder of Mrs. Crippen. The case is interesting in that no body was found, and the case hinged on the fact that the tissue discovered was found to contain the toxic alkaloidal compound hyoscine, which had not been known ever to have been used in a poisoning homicide up to that time. It was also proven that Dr. Crippen had purchased hyoscine, to use—he claimed—in the preparation of his homeopathic formulations. Ethel Le Neve was found not guilty of any involvement in the death of Mrs. Crippen, but Dr. Crippen was found guilty, and was hanged on November 23, 1910. Many books have been written on the Crippen murder, and the name "Crippen" has even become a synonym for poisoner in the British language. Many students of the case have asked why he did not simply walk away from his unhappy marriage in the first place. Also, why did he dismember Cora's body, which certainly did not point to a natural death. Hyoscine was used at the time, in certain institutions, for a sedative effect. It is possible he gave her the hyoscine to depress her sexual appetite, since he might have found it difficult to be sexually involved with two women at the same time, and accidentally overdosed her. Perhaps he had shot her, as there was a gun in the home (which never came out at the trial), and then realized he had to get rid of the body. We probably will never have the true answers to these questions. But Crippen and Le Neve have been immortalized in wax in Madame Tussaud's Waxworks' "Chamber of Horrors" in London, for all visitors to look upon their visages and wonder.

1.2.8. Frederick Seddon, "The Poisoning Miser" (1911)

Frederick Seddon was a miser. In an attempt to gain easier access to the financial assets of another person, he took a boarder named Elizabeth Barrow in to his London home. Frederick soon convinced the woman to assign him controlling interest in her annuities, in exchange for a promise to care for her for the rest of her life. After several episodes of severe stomach distress, Elizabeth died in the Seddon home on September 14, 1911. Suspicious relatives soon arrived to take possession of the dead woman's estate, and were told by Seddon that there was nothing left to turn over. They went to the police with their suspicions, and it was soon determined that the victim's body contained massive amounts of arsenic. Frederick and his wife Mary became prime suspects in her untimely death. It was proven that Mary Seddon had purchased a large number of insecticidal fly papers, which contained arsenic, and it was speculated that the deadly poison had been soaked from the product and given to the deceased. Mary was eventually found innocent of any crime, but Frederick was found guilty and was hanged on April 18, 1912.

1.2.9. Henri Girard, "The First Scientific Murderer" (1912)

This case is important in our collection as it represents one of the first known uses of biological agents to carry out a poisoning homicide. The financial manipulator, Mr. Girard, purportedly a rather dashing-looking Parisian, made it his practice to insure the lives of various acquaintances having himself listed as their prime beneficiary. These people soon died under mysterious circumstances by the hand of their friend. Girardi's poisonous weapons of choice were the natural toxins from the mushrooms of genus *Amanita*, as well as various pathogenic bacteria. Soon after the deaths of Girard's acquaintances, Louis Pernotte and Madame Monin, the insurance companies became very suspicious, and an investigation ensued. Girard was taken into custody in 1912, but cheated the French court by taking one of his own toxic germ cultures (most likely typhoid), which he had secreted in his personal effects.

1.2.10. Arthur Warren Waite, DDS, "The Playboy Poisoner" (1916)

The first dentist in our collection, Dr. Waite, was a good looking raconteur, who most likely preferred playing tennis to practicing dentistry. He grew up in Grand Rapids, Michigan, and after graduating from dental school went to South Africa to practice. Waite eventually left Africa under some suspicious accusations and returned to Michigan, where he wooed and married the daughter of John and Hannah Peck. John Peck was a millionaire pharmacist who owned a reputable drug company in the city. The newlyweds were furnished with posh accommodations in New York City by the grateful Pecks. There, Arthur spent much of his time dabbling in the area of bacteriology, and also took on a mistress. In January 1916, shortly after Hannah Peck arrived to visit the Waites in New York, she suddenly became ill and died. Her body was immediately cremated and returned to Michigan for burial. In March of the same year, John Peck also went to New York to console his daughter and her husband over the death of his wife. He too soon became ill and died. However, before his body could be cremated an anonymous telegram was received in Grand Rapids stating "suspicion aroused, demand autopsy." Surprisingly, the autopsy indicated that John Peck was loaded with arsenic, and an investigation ensued. The accusing finger eventually pointed to the playboy dentist, and he was taken in for interrogation. A search of his dwelling revealed numerous bacterial cultures, as well as texts dealing with toxicology. Under interrogation, Dr. Waite changed his story numerous times. First he stated that he had obtained arsenic for his father-in-law, who wanted to commit suicide to end his grief over the loss of his wife. Then Dr. Waite claimed his own body was inhabited by the spirit of an evil Egyptian priest, who had instructed him to kill his in-laws in order to gain their wealth. Eventually, Dr. Waite felt if he told what had actually happened the courts would find him insane, so he revealed the whole story of administering typhoid, pneumonia, diphtheria organisms, and arsenic while the Peck's were undergoing work in his dental chair. It did not take the jury long to see through the manipulations of Dr. Waite, and they convicted him of the murders. Dr. Waite was electrocuted at Sing Sing Prison on May 24, 1917.

1.2.11. Murderers of Mike Malloy, "The Case of the Man Who Wouldn't Die" (1933)

This is a rare case of multiple offenders on a single victim, which, in retrospect, is almost humorous in some respects. In January 1933, New York City and the rest of America were in the middle of the Great Depression. A group of men in a bar devised a way to make some easy money, by insuring the life of someone and then murdering him to collect on the policy. Dan Kreigsberg, a local grocer; David "Red" Murphy, a barman; Anthony "Tony" Marino, the bar owner; and Frank Pasqua, an undertaker, chose as their patsy a well-known Irish alcoholic and "skid-row" resident named Mike Malloy, who happened to come through the door of the establishment. After the $1600 policy was initiated, they soon began to offer Malloy free drinks and food, which he thought was very generous from his new friends. However, along with the pure alcohol he was being given, the plotters added horse liniment, and sometimes antifreeze to his drinks. The food was filled with carpet tacks and other potentially harmful foreign bodies. Unfortunately for the group, Malloy seemed to ingest these substances with little harm. Becoming desperate, they then got Malloy drunk and threw him out into a park in the middle of a winter storm, hoping that the temperature would do the job. The next day, their victim returned for more of their hospitality.

The group then retained the services of a taxi driver, and, after standing the drunken man up in the middle of the street, he was struck by the moving taxi. He survived this encounter too. Feeling that were having to work too hard for their money, the group decided to carry out the murder once and for all. They took the drunken Malloy to his bedroom, ran a hose from the gas light on the wall down his throat, and killed him with coal gas. They collected their insurance money, and all would have gone well if one of the group had not bragged about their project. When the police were informed, the entire group were placed on trial for the crime. The outcome was not what the group had envisioned when they started out on their money-making scheme: the four were electrocuted on June 8, 1934 for the crime. Hersey Green, the taxi driver, received a prison sentence.

1.2.12. Rev. Frank Elias Sipple, "The Poisoning Pastor" (1939)

Sometimes even a minister can be a poisoner. In 1939, in Grand Rapids, Michigan, the Reverend Frank Sipple was a spiritual leader of the Southlawn Church of God. He decided to murder his daughter, Dorothy Ann, and gave her a capsule containing cyanide. The act was carried out one Sunday morning just before he left for the church to deliver his weekly sermon. Death examiners missed the true cause of the girl's death, and she was buried without further investigation. The homicide remained undetected until 1946, when Pastor Sipple attacked one of the church elder's with a lead pipe. The gentleman who had been the target of the pastor's attack also claimed he thought the minister had once given him candies that had been tampered with. Under interrogation by the police, Sipple admitted not only to the attack on the parishioner, but also to the poisoning death of his daughter many years earlier. The suspect stated his daughter was mentally disturbed and he thought she would be better dead than having to spend her life in a mental institution. There was some speculation that his daughter might have had some information on the untimely death of Frank's first wife, and was possibly going to take the matter to the local authorities. The court found Rev. Sipple guilty of murder and he was sentenced to life in prison. Ill with terminal cancer, he was eventually released from prison to return to Grand Rapids, where he soon died.

1.2.13. Sadamichi Hirasawa, "The Poisoning Bank Robber" (1948)

On January 26, 1949, a mass killer with a most unique plan struck at the suburban Shiinamaki branch of the Teikoku Imperial Bank in Tokyo, Japan. Sadamichi Hirasawa, pretending to be a Dr. Jiro Yamaguchi, entered the bank's facility at closing time, telling the 14 bank employees that they must drink some medicine to prevent an outbreak of amoebic dysentery then rampant in the district. The employees obediently swallowed teacups full of a liquid heavily laced with the deadly poison, potassium cyanide. Thirteen of the bank's employees died on the spot, upon which Hirasawa looted the bank of more than 180,000 yen (then about $600) and vanished into the general population. In one of the largest manhunts in Japanese history, the police laboriously interviewed thousands of people who had received business cards from a man pretending to be a physician, and finally pinpointed Hirasawa. An artist, Sadamichi was identified by the lone surviving bank employee, admitted his guilt, and was imprisoned for life. After spending 40 years on death row, he died in 1987, gaining some international fame as the longest resident on death row anywhere in the world. Recently there has been some speculation that Sadamichi might have been innocent of the robbery, and that the crime was actually carried out by a renegade member of the Japanese Army's disbanded, and very secret, "Unit 731," that during World War II had carried out bacteriological research experiments on human prisoners of war in Manchuria.

1.2.14. Christa Ambros Lehmann, "The Poisonous Neighbor" (1954)

The Lehmann case is interesting because of the relatively common background of the poisoner and the poison she selected. In February, 1954, in the town of Worms, Germany, Christa purchased five chocolate truffle candies at a local shop, and delivered four of them to her friends, keeping one candy as a special gift for a woman who had been objecting to Christa's association with members of the woman's family. The targeted victim, instead of eating the candy, placed it in a kitchen cupboard as a treat for her daughter to eat. When the daughter sampled the treat, she complained of the bitter taste and dropped it on the floor, where it was quickly consumed by the family dog. Within a short time, both the girl and the pet were dead, and the attending physician was somewhat puzzled by the common symptoms and sudden fatalities exhibited by the two victims. Eventually the cause of the deaths was traced to a relatively new chemical substance called *E-605*, which had been developed as a potent insecticide. We now know this substance as Parathion, which acts much like a nerve-gas agent, causing rapid alterations in the victim's autonomic nervous system, leading to death with a characteristic set of symptoms. Suspicion fell immediately on Christa as the provider of the candy, and during her police interrogation, she confessed to using *E-605* as the poisoning agent. While in police custody, she also admitted to killing her husband and her father-in-law with the same toxic compound. The court sentenced her to life in prison. Unfortunately, the discussion of the poison and its potential in the press soon led to a rash of *E-605* suicides in Germany among individuals depressed over the state of post-war Germany.

1.2.15. Arthur Kendrick Ford, "The Accidental Poisoner for Sex" (1954)

This case illustrates that not all poisonings are murder in the first degree. Arthur Ford was infatuated with two female coworkers in his London chemical company, and decided he needed some chemical assistance in gaining their sexual attentions. Having heard about the effects of "Spanish Fly" as an aphrodisiac, he obtained the natural form of Cantharides from the firm's stockroom, stating that he needed it to breed rabbits. On April 27, 1954, Arthur entered the company's office and offered three of the secretaries some coconut candies in which he had placed large doses of the powdered Cantharide. Neither he nor the unfortunate women knew the horrible physical torment they would soon endure. Cantharidin, which is derived from the ground-up bodies of a Mediterranean beetle, is a powerful blistering agent normally used in dermatology to burn off warts. The corrosive effect of this compound on the human anatomy is disastrous. After only a few hours, all three women were hospitalized in torment, and two of them died from the ill effects. When autopsies revealed the cause of the deaths, Ford broke down upon being interviewed and confessed to his involvement. He was placed on trial, and—because it was not his intent to murder—he was convicted of manslaughter and sentenced to five years in prison.

1.2.16. Nannie ("Arsenic Annie") Doss, "The Poisonous Romantic" (1954)

Nannie Doss was a female serial killer, if there ever was one. By the time she was finally detected, she had successfully poisoned a total of eleven victims, including five husbands, two children, her mother, two sisters, and a nephew. Nannie was a housewife, living in Tulsa, Oklahoma, and first came to the attention of the local authorities in 1954, when a suspicious physician decided to autopsy her deceased fifth husband. The analysis revealed an amount of arsenic equal to 20 lethal doses. The exhumation and toxicological analyses of other members of her family who had died over the years also revealed the presence of arsenic. Upon interrogation, her crimes came to light, and she stated that she had done away with her husbands because she had found them to be dull. This was probably related to the fact that Nannie's favorite reading material consisted of romance magazines, and her domestic life had not measured up to her romantic fantasies. Found guilty of the multiple murders, she was sentenced to life in prison, where she died from leukemia in 1965.

1.2.17. Graham Frederick Young, "The Toxicomaniac" (1971)

Perhaps one of the most fascinating of the poisoner personalities is represented by an Englishman named Graham Young: he was a "toxicomaniac," or a lover of poisons. The poisons gave him a feeling of power over other people, and he used poisons throughout his life to nefarious ends. At the age of 11 years, his father gave him a chemistry set for his birthday, and from that time on Graham followed his obsession with chemistry and toxicology. He read incessantly about the crimes of the infamous poisoners, and became very conversant with the subject of poisons. He once told his sister that he would become more famous than the well-known British poisoners Palmer, Pritchard, and Crippen. Graham's stepmother died when he was 14 years old, and no one suspected that he had played a key role in her death by the administration of an antimony-containing compound. Other members of his immediate family, as well as school friends, also became subjects for his toxicological experiments. In 1962, when one of his teachers accidentally found strange notes and drawings in Graham's school desk, the authorities were called in to investigate. In his room at home, they found enough various poisons to kill almost 300 people, along with an extensive reference library on poisons. He was remanded to Broadmoor Criminal Lunatic Asylum, a mental facility, until it was determined he was cured of his abnormal psychological affliction. Deemed rehabilitated by the asylum's psychologists, he was released after a period of only nine years.

In 1971, Graham began working at a photographic optical firm in Bovington, England, which specialized in the production of high-quality optical lenses. In the production of these lenses, the company utilized the deadly poisonous element thallium, which coincidentally happened to be one of Graham's favorite poisonous tools. One of his jobs at the facility was passing out the daily tea on breaks. A wave of illness soon spread throughout the company, and two of his coworkers died from a supposed viral nervous system illness. When the company doctor was called in to address the concerns of the employees over what had become known as the "Bovington Bug," Graham drew attention to himself by freely spouting his knowledge of toxicology, and why he felt the physicians had missed in their diagnosis of a viral cause. He said that they failed to see that the symptoms were much more consistent with thallium poisoning. A review of Graham's past soon revealed he had been hospitalized for his poison mania, and a search warrant was obtained for his lodgings. In his room the investigators found a diary that revealed the names of the individuals he had selected for his toxicological experiments, and notations on the effects of the administered poisons over the course of their intoxications. While awaiting trial Graham boasted that he had committed the perfect crime in 1962, in the killing and subsequent cremation of his stepmother. In June 1972, Graham was found guilty of two murders, two attempted murders, and two charges of administering poisons, and was sentenced to life in prison. In 1990, at age 42, Graham died in prison from a heart attack, thus, ending the life of one of the most cruel, yet forensically fascinating, poisoning personalities yet known.

1.2.18. Ronald Clark O'Bryan, "The Halloween Killer" (1974)

Poisoners are despised by the public for their lack of sympathy toward their victim, and rightly so in the case of Ronald Clark O'Bryan, who killed his own child to obtain money from an insurance policy. On October 31, 1974, in the town of Pasadena, Texas, eight-year-old Timothy Marc O'Bryan died after ingesting a Halloween treat. Examination of the candy straws filled with fruit-flavored powder called "Pixy Stix®," revealed that it also contained potassium cyanide. Contaminated treats were also found in the candy bags of other children from the neighborhood. Mr. O'Bryan, who had accompanied the children around the neighborhood on their trick-or-treat activities, stated that the poisoned candies had been given out from the home of a rather shadowy figure he could not identify. Police investigation eventually revealed that the 30-year-old O'Bryan had made inquiries around his workplace concerning cyanide, and had recently taken out a $65,000 insurance policy on his son. The court found him guilty of the murder, and he was executed—ironically, by lethal injection—on March 31, 1984.

1.2.19. Rev. James Warren Jones, "The Minister Who Went Mad" (1978)

Many people can easily remember the television news scenes of November 18, 1978 showing 913 people lying dead in the sun in a jungle compound in the South American country of Guyana. This case represents one of the greatest mass suicides (murders?) involving poison in recent history. The pivotal personality involved in this incident, Reverend Jim Jones, did not administer the poison with his own hands, but he certainly was the instigating force in this terrible event. Jones, who founded a communal group known as the "People's Temple," had taken his flock to the jungles of Guyana and founded a spiritual refuge known as "Jonestown."

Jones was a prime example of the famous quote by Lord Acton, that power corrupts, and absolute power corrupts absolutely. In Guyana, Jones eventually lost touch with reality, becoming extremely paranoid in his view of the outside world. The triggering event to the mass poisoning was the visit of California Congressman Leo Ryan to investigate allegations made by the families of some of his constituents about Jones' hold over members of their families. Congressman Ryan, and many other members of his entourage, were shot and killed at Jonestown by Jones' followers, and then Jim Jones ordered his followers to carry out the "white night" exercises they had practiced so many times as a test of their faith for their pastoral leader. A large container of fruit drink containing cyanide and sedatives was soon concocted, and many of the people lined up and voluntarily drank the deadly creation. Some, however, were less than willing to die for Jones' cause; many of the bodies bore signs that the poison had been injected by force. Jones' body was also recovered from the commune death scene, but the cause of his death was a bullet to the head. A review of this terrible tragedy in Guyana reminds one of the Euripides saying that, "whom the gods destroy, they first make mad."

1.2.20. Murder of Georgi Markov, "The Umbrella Assassination" (1978)

Murdering a victim by means of poison can also be a political act. The Markov case represents a most unique murder with poison, because of the means of administration. Georgi Markov was a Bulgarian defector living in London and working for the BBC, broadcasting pro-Western propoganda materials back to his Communist-controlled homeland. While going to work on the morning of September 7, 1978, Markov felt a stabbing pain in his thigh, and a man in the crowd behind him suddenly dropped and then quickly picked up an umbrella. The unknown man apologized for bumping into him, then entered a taxicab and disappeared. Over the next several days, Markov became increasingly ill, and medical teams were unable to discover the cause of his symptoms and of the changes that were happening to his normal blood constituents. Within four days of the event, Markov was dead. An autopsy of the victim revealed a small bruise mark on his thigh, which, when excised, revealed a pin-head sized metal sphere with holes drilled into it. Although no poison could be detected in this metal object, the toxicologists generally agreed that the poison that induced Markov's symptoms was most likely ricin, a highly toxic plant substance found in the castor bean (*Ricinus communis L.*). Georgi Markov's assassin was never found, and after the fall of the Soviet Union, it was revealed that ricin was indeed used in an umbrella mechanism for the means of injecting the poisoned spheres into their victim. The case, bought by Markov's widow, is currently in the courts.

1.2.21. Unknown Offender, "The Tylenol® Tamperer" (1982)

In October, 1982, a series of incidents occurred in Chicago that were to change forever the manner in which over-the-counter (OTC) medication was to be sold in the United States. Seven people were to fall victim to a tamperer when they innocently took Extra Strength Tylenol® capsules that had been laced with cyanide. Of the seven victims, six died almost immediately, and one lived for two days before succumbing to the effects of the poison. It took some time before investigators were able to determine that the common factor in all the deaths was that all seven victims had taken the pain reliever. As a result of this incident, the product's manufacturer immediately recalled all packages of their analgesic product on a national level, and reformulated both the capsule format and packaging to make them more tamper-resistant. In their prompt attention to the problem, the company was able to save their credibility with the public, and set a standard for other manufacturers on handling any similar future incidents. Although an extensive investigation ensued, there was never sufficient evidence obtained to warrant the arrest of an individual for this heinous crime. As a result of this incident, tamper-resistant packaging has became a norm in the American marketplace.

1.2.22. Stella Maudine Nickell, "The Camouflaged Poisoner" (1986)

In poisoning cases, things are not always as they first appear. The case of Stella Nickell is a perfect example of what appeared to be a death resulting from a tampering incident, but was actually an attempt to cover up a very carefully planned out homicide.

In Auburn, Washington, Nickell's husband, Bruce, died from what was believed to be emphysema. The cause of his death was actually the effects of cyanide, which had been administered by his wife in an attempt to collect on a life insurance policy. Unfortunately for Stella Nickell, a natural cause of death did not pay as much as an accidental death. Out of this dilemma, she concocted a plan.

Not long after, a young woman named Susan Snow collapsed and died in the bathroom of her own home, after taking an over-the-counter pain reliever. Upon autopsy, cyanide was detected in the unfortunate woman. An investigation of her movements just before her death lead to the discovery of a bottle of pain reliever capsules in her medicine cabinet that had been tampered with, and cyanide was found as the tampering agent. A rapidly instituted recall by the product's manufacturer revealed several other bottles of tampered medication in different locations. The case took an interesting turn when Nickell called the authorities to report that she thought her husband had also been a victim of this tainted pain reliever. Exhumation revealed that Bruce had also died from cyanide poisoning, and two bottles of contaminated capsules were found in the Nickell home. Stella said that she had purchased these bottles at two different stores, and it didn't take the authorities long to realize that they were either talking to the most unlucky purchaser in history, or to someone who might know more about this tampering incident then it first appeared. Evidence began to mount against Stella, and suspicions were voiced by other members of her family. In addition, authorities found small green flecks of material in the cyanide, which was eventually identified as an algae destroyer used in home aquariums. The Nickell's home contained many such aquariums. A forensic investigation of books at the local library eventually revealed many of Stella's fingerprints on toxicology books dealing with cyanide and other toxic compounds. The jury found Stella guilty of two murders, and she was sentenced to two 90-year terms in prison.

1.2.23. Donald Harvey, "The Angel of Death" (1983–1987)

Here we have the case of a serial killer who struck at victims within the health care system over a period of four years, from 1983 to 1987. Donald Harvey, a nurse's aide, used multiple methods to bring the lives of many patients under his care to a rapid end. Some were smothered, and some he poisoned with arsenic or cyanide. His crimes eventually came to light in Cincinnati, Ohio, when a pathologist was able to detect the odor of cyanide on one of the hospital victims he legally had to autopsy. Further exhumations and autopsies were performed on other patients who had died unexpectedly during a given time period, and traces of poison were found in many of the bodies. One of the common factors shared by these victims was that they were cared for by Donald Harvey. Upon interrogation, Harvey admitted to the killings, and was placed on trial. It was determined by court psychiatrists that Harvey had a personality disorder that resulted in a compulsion to kill, but was not insane. After pleading guilty to 24 murders, Donald Harvey was sentenced to three consecutive life terms in prison. Thus was incarcerated one of the most prolific medical poisoners in the history of the United States.

1.2.24. George Trepal, "The Eccentric Genius" (1988)

George Trepal was probably one of the most intelligent poisoners ever encountered in the United States. His IQ qualified him for membership in *Mensa*, a select group of individuals with proven high intelligence, representing probably only 2% of the general population.

The case began in 1988, in Bartow, Florida, when several members of the Carr family suddenly became ill. Something unknown was causing paralysis and slow destruction of their nervous systems. Thought to be the result of a virus, they were hospitalized and provided whatever supportive care was possible. Eventually the mother of the family, Peggy Carr, succumbed from her condition, and one of her sons was permanently disabled by the effects on his nervous system. Suspicion fell on the heavy metal poison thallium as the cause of the family's maladies, and a search began for a possible environmental source of the substance. Investigation finally settled on the presence of the element in bottles of Coca Cola® that the family had consumed over a period of time. The question was, how did this very toxic substance wind up in this consumer product? Obviously someone had tampered with the bottles. During the extensive investigation, the person who came to light was a neighbor, who had openly voiced some displeasure with the members of the Carr family over various neighborhood issues. An undercover police investigation revealed that Trepal had had access to the family, a motive, and a great deal of knowledge about chemistry. A search of his home revealed a container with traces of thallium. Trepal was found guilty of the tampering murder, and was sentenced to die for the crime. At the time of this writing, he is awaiting execution on death row in Florida.

1.3. CONCLUSION

This chapter is but a brief overview of a few of the more infamous people who chose to use poison as their weapon to achieve nefarious ends. We can only imagine the hundreds of individuals who have also used such a weapon, and whose crimes have gone undetected.

To read more about infamous poisoners, the author recommends the concise work by Michael Farrell, cited in the Suggested Readings list.

1.4. REFERENCES

Beerbohm M: *And Even Now,* William Heinemann, London, 1920.

Bombaugh CC: Female poisoners: ancient and modern. *Johns Hopkins Hospital–Bulletin,* 1899;101–102:148–153.

Meek WJ: The gentle art of poisoning. *Phi Beta Pi Quarterly,* May, 1928.

Osius TG: The historic art of poisoning. *Univ. of Michigan Medical Bulletin,* 1957;23(3):111–116.

Smith S: Poisons and poisoners through the ages. *Medico-Legal Journal,* 1952; 20:153–166.

1.5. SUGGESTED READINGS

Bagchi KN: *Poisons and Poisoning: Their History and Romance and Their Detection in Crimes.* Kshentamani-Nagendralal Memorial Lectures for 1964, University of Calcutta, Calcutta, India, 1969.

Cabannes A, and Nass L: *Poisons et sortileges* [Poisons and Spells], Parts I & II. Librarie Plon, Paris, France, 1903 [in French].

Farrell M: *Poisons and Poisoners: An Encyclopedia of Homicidal Poisonings.* Robert Hale, London, 1992.

Lewin L: *Die Gifte in der Weltgeschichte* [Poisons in World History]. Verlag Von Julius Springer, Berlin, Germany, 1920 [in German].

Mangin A: *Le Poisons* [Poisons]. Alfred Mame & Sons, Tours, France, 1869 [in French].

Nash JR: *Encyclopedia of World Crime.* Crime Books, Inc., Wilmette, IL, 1990.

Thompson CJS: *Poison Romance and Poison Mysteries.* The Scientific Press Ltd., London, 1899.

Thompson CJS: *Poison Mysteries in History, Romance, and Crime.* J.B. Lippincott, Philadelphia, 1924.

Thompson CJS: *Poisons and Poisoners—With Some Historical Accounts of Some Famous Mysteries in Ancient and Modern Times,* Harold Shaylor, London, 1931.

Thompson CJS: *Poison Mysteries Unsolved: "By Person or Persons Unknown,"* Hutchinson & Co., London, 1937.

Chapter 2

Types of Poisons

> *"Poisons and medicines are oftentimes the same substance given with different intents."* —Peter Mere Latham

In this chapter we will discuss the nuances of poison as a weapon. What is a poison? What advantages does this type of weapon offer over the more traditional types of death-inflicting instruments?

2.1. DEFINITIONS

At the outset it might seem simple enough to define what a poison is; however, legally it is not quite as simple as it first appears. In the courts the definition of "poison" has oftentimes been difficult to agree upon. *Scientific American* once humorously defined a poison as,

> *"any substance in relatively small quantities that can cause death or illness in living organisms by chemical action. The qualification 'by chemical action,' is necessary because it rules out such effects as those produced by a small quantity of lead entering the body at high velocity."*

Humor aside, in the courtroom a great deal of discussion will ensue concerning whether the substance in question is really a poison. Is aspirin a poison? Most would agree that it is a medicinal agent, because people take this substance to relieve pain and fever. However, in sufficient dosages aspirin can be an agent that results in death. So what is a poison? Although definitions may differ according to the laws of various states, to follow are some of the definitions of poison that have been cited in the legal literature:

> *" POISON: is any substance, where introduced into the system, either directly or by absorption, produces violent, morbid or fatal changes, or which destroys living tissue with which it comes in contact." (Watkins v. National Elec. Products Corp.,* C.C.A. Pa., 165, F.2d 980, 982)

> *"POISON: Any substance which, when relatively small amounts are ingested, inhaled, or absorbed, or applied to, injected into, or developed within the body, has chemical action that may cause damage to structure or disturbance of function producing symptomology, illness, or death." (Stedman's Medical Dictionary,* 26th ed., Williams & Wilkins, Baltimore, MD, 1995)

> *"POISON: Any substance which, when ingested, inhaled, or absorbed, or when applied to, injected into, or developed within the body, in relatively small amounts, by its chemical action may cause damage to structure or disturbance of function." (The Sloane-Dorland Annotated Medical-Legal Dictionary,* West Publishing Co., New York, NY, 1987)

Probably the most astute concept of what constitutes the difference between a poisonous and a nonpoisonous substance was stated by the famous 16th century alchemist Philippus Aureolus Theophrastus Bombastus von Hohenheim-Paracelsus (1493–1541), when he wrote:

> *"What is there that is not poison, all things are poison and nothing (is) without poison. Solely the dose determines that a thing is not a poison."*

In this statement, Paracelsus was able to get to the very core of the argument of what determines, or defines, a poison; which is that anything can be a poison—it merely depends on what dose causes deleterious effects. Certainly the relaxation that might come from drinking a relatively small amount of an alcoholic beverage, when compared to a death that may result from ethanol intoxication (as experienced by a fraternity initiation, for example) is merely dose-related outcome. The same principle applies to the medications we routinely take to keep our bodies in healthy balance. Toxicology is nothing more than the subject of pharmacology (the study of the actions of drugs), pushed too far, into the "dark side" as it were.

2.2. CHARACTERISTICS OF "IDEAL" POISONS

There are certain characteristics that characterize an "ideal" poison, and the homicidal poisoner will select their murderous compounds to encompass as many of these characteristics as possible. What follows are some of the characteristics of an "ideal" homicidal poison:

- It should be odorless, tasteless, and colorless, as this allows for administration to the intended victim, providing no warning signs that the victim can detect by the normal bodily senses of smell, taste, and sight.
- It should be readily soluble, preferably in water, as this allows for easy administration in normal foods and drinks that the victim may partake.
- It should have a delayed onset of action, as this allows for a time period in which the poisoner can attempt to create an alibi.
- It should be undetectable, and certainly the more exotic the poison the more likely that it will not be detected in more routine toxicological analyses.
- It should have a low-dose lethality, which means less of the toxic material needs to be administered in the dose. It is much easier to administer a pinch of a substance, rather than a pound.
- It should be easily obtained, but not traceable, so it will leave no investigative trail that would lead to the poisoner.
- It should be chemically stable, which makes it easy to store without loss of potency.

The heavy metals (e.g., arsenic, antimony, mercury, lead, etc.) are elements or elemental compounds, and are as toxic today as they were when first created millions of years ago. This can also be an advantage for law enforcement investigator, as these compounds tend to remain detectable many years after burial of the victim.

Probably one of the greatest things desired is for the poison to mimic a natural disease state, as the poisoning will be missed. A death certificate would then bear an unrelated medical cause of death, and the victim would be buried without detection of an actual crime.

Table 2-1
"Ideal" Poison Characteristics

Tasteless
Odorless
Colorless
Readily soluble
Delayed onset of action
Undetectable
Exotic
Low-dose lethality
Easily obtained (not traceable)
Chemically stable
Mimics a natural disease

These ideal characteristics are summarized in **Table 2-1.**

2.3. CONTRASTS BETWEEN POISONS AND MORE TRADITIONAL WEAPONS

Certainly one of the main advantages enjoyed by poison over the more traditional weapons is that it is invisible as a weapon. One might therefore consider it a "stealth" weapon. The unsuspecting victim never sees it coming and therefore can not put up any form of reasonable defense to the attack.

In effect, a poison is a "chemical bomb," which does not explode with an external violent force, but nonetheless, like an explosive, destroys the internal natural workings of the victim's physiology. It could be reasonably hypothesized, therefore, that a poisoner would show some of the same characteristics one would find in the profile of a bomber. Common characteristics of a bomber include: Caucasian; male; average to above average intelligence; underachiever; inadequate personality; nonathletic; cowardly; neat and orderly; meticulous; loner; careful planner; and nonconfrontational (either physically or psychologically).

There usually is no trauma or visible signs of the poison's effects on the victim's body, as the body kills itself physiologically via a chemical short circuit. This allows the poisoner to design the symptoms exhibited by the victim, by the chemical and toxicological nature of the poison selected. The victim has no protection as long as he eats, drinks, and breaths. Of course, if the poisoner could get the victim to stop these essential natural body processes, there would be no need to administer the poison. However, since we must all constantly carry out the processes of eating, drinking, and breathing, we are all essentially constantly vulnerable to the attack of the poisoner.

A poison is a silent weapon. There is no noise like a gun, therefore a poison could be considered the ultimate silencer. Unlike a gunshot, it is doubtful that a witness could be obtained who could state that they heard the sound of a cyanide molecule going off in the dead of the night that awoke everyone in the dwelling. In an attack carried out with a gun, there is always the chance that some innocent bystander could become injured or killed. However, poison allows the careful-planning poisoner to carry out very precise targeting on the victim, leaving nearby bystanders unaware that the crime has even been attempted or perpetrated. Thus, for a very good poisoner, it is possible to murder a single individual at large banquet, although this would necessitate a great deal of planning and access.

Certainly a poison allows the poisoner to overcome easily a physically or mentally stronger person by invading their defense zone. The poisoner may be physically or psychologically nonconfrontational. In this manner, a petite wife can easily overcome the brute strength of an abusive spouse. At the same time, a weaker-willed husband could overcome the abusive personality of a more domineering wife.

If the first attempt is to poison is unsuccessful, this type of weapon provides a chance for the poisoner to try again, as the victim is still unaware that an initial attempt at murder has even been made.

Unlike with more traditional weapons, the poisoner is unlikely to be disarmed and have his weapon used against him.

As a poison, the weapon is very easily overlooked at the death (crime) scene, as it will often appear like any natural substance that is usually found in the environment.

With this type of weapon, it is very possible to make a murder look like suicide, or make a suicide look like murder.

For the poisoner who might be squeamish at the site of blood or gore, or is concerned about having to clean up the death scene of the murder, there is no such messy component to this crime.

With this type of murder, there is a certain degree of depersonalization, as in the mind of the poisoner he merely sets the trap, but the victim actually springs it. This attempts to rationalize, and to lessen the guilt that

Table 2-2
Poison Advantages Over Other Weapons

Invisible weapon (stealth-like)
Chemical bomb
Body kills itself physiologically
No protection (we all must eat, drink, and breathe)
No noise (a supreme silencer)
No gore for the squeamish
Depersonalization (only setting the trap)
If unsuccessful, the poisoner can try again
Precise targeting
Easy to overcome a stronger person

the poisoner may feel by being the one who actively pulls the trigger of a gun or plunges a knife. These advantages are summarized in **Table 2.2.**

2.4. HOW DO POISONS KILL?

Like a wrench thrown into the finely tuned engine of a car would disrupt its proper running, the chemical molecule, like a "chemical monkey wrench," disrupts the proper running of the body's biochemical processes. There are literally thousands of these "chemical monkey wrenches" available to the poisoner. Each poison can be carefully selected to disrupt a specific body process.

Some of the major classifications of poisons based upon how they will do their dirty work on various organ system can be seen in **Table 2-3.**

Poisons can kill the victim in a number of ways, depending on the effects of the chemical substance on the body's normal physiology.

2.4.1. Central Nervous System (CNS) Effects

By altering the critical function of the body's nervous system, the poison can cause central nervous system depression, resulting in coma; loss of the respiratory drive, resulting in the stoppage of breathing (respiratory arrest); loss of the reflexes protecting the airway, resulting in the flaccid tongue obstructing the airway, or aspiration of gastric contents into the bronchial tree. The poison can also affect the heart with cardiovascular (circulatory) effects, including hypotension (low blood pressure) from decreased cardiac contractions, hypovolemia from loss of fluids, peripheral vascular collapse, or cardiac arrhythmias.

The body's cells can die from a lack of oxygen necessary for normal cellular respirations, called cellular hypoxia (lack of oxygen), owing to

Table 2-3
"Chemical Monkey Wrench" Targets

Cause	Effect
Irritant chemicals (e.g., acids)	Inflammation
Heavy metals (e.g., arsenic, antimony, lead, thallium)	Enzyme inhibition
Atropine, botulism, hyoscyamine, strychnine	Receptor-site interference (ANS, CNS, and other sites
Chemicals (e.g., sodium monofluoroacetate)	Lethal synthesis
Chemicals (e.g., fungal amatoxins, paraquat, acetaminophen)	Essential organ necrosis
Chemicals (e.g., carbon tetrachloride)	Lipid peroxidation
Carcinogenic chemicals (e.g., Benzene)	Neoplasia
Multiple chemical substances	Miscellaneous pharmacological effects

a breakdown in the normal transport of oxygen. There can be seizures resulting from muscle hyperactivity, which results in hyperpyrexia (increase in body temperature), or kidney failure, resulting from destruction of muscle tissue (deposition of myoglobin in the kidneys). There can be brain damage from lack of oxygen, which results in the loss of the master control for the entire body engine. Death can result from pulmonary aspiration, resulting in chemically induced pneumonia and destruction of the lungs.

Some poisons seem to pinpoint specifically a particular body vital organ, such as the lung destruction caused by the herbicide Paraquat, the destruction of the liver caused by the analgesic acetaminophen (APAP) or the fungal amatoxins, or the destruction of the kidneys caused by antifreeze (ethylene glycol), or another fungal toxin called orellanine.

Poison profiles for the investigating officer and analytical toxicologist, for some of the more common homicidal poisons, can be found in the Appendix to this work. In each profile, the investigator will find discussions of the following important points about the poison:

1. Form.
2. Common color.
3. Characteristic odors.

4. Solubility.
5. Taste.
6. Common sources.
7. Lethal dose.
8. Mechanism.
9. Possible methods of administration.
10. Time interval of onset of symptoms.
11. Symptoms resulting from an acute exposure.
12. Symptoms resulting from chronic exposure.
13. Disease states mimicked by poisoning.
14. Notes relating to the victim.
15. Specimens from victim to be obtained for analysis.
16. Analytical detection methods.
17. Known toxic levels.
18. Notes pertinent to analysis of the poison.
19. List of selected homicide cases in which particular poisons have been used.

What quantity a poison would be necessary to produce a lethal outcome in a human victim? Many individuals are surprised to learn that a minute amount of a poison can result in death. To give the reader a hands-on feel for lethal amounts, let us use as a reference the weight of a US dime. The average American dime weighs approximately 2600 mg. If one had the same weight of some common homicidal poison equivalent to coin, how many human lethal doses would this weight equal? *See* **Table 2-4.**

2.4.2. Other Categories of Poisons

Poisons as weapons contain a lot of "molecular firepower." When one pulls the trigger on a gun, one in effect releases a single piece of lead that the offender hopes will produce a lethal effect on the intended target, by disrupting body tissue and vital organs that will lead to the target's death. However, with a poison, one does not unleash a single bullet, but literally millions of chemical bullets, to do their lethal business. How many chemical molecules are contained in a lethal dose? With an elementary knowledge of chemical principles, one can easily calculate the number of "killer molecules" contained in a lethal dose of any substance. This calculation is based on what is known as "Avogadro's Number," which states that there are 6.02×10^{23} molecules, or atoms, per gram molecular weight (GMW) of any substance.

Table 2-4
Poison Lethal Doses in the Weight of a Dime

Poison	Lethal Dose(LD)	#LDs
Thallium	1,000 mg	2
Compound "1080"	700 mg	3
Cyanide	200 mg	13
Arsenic	200 mg	13
Strychnine	100 mg	26
Botulinus toxin	50 ng	52,000,000

If one then takes the minimum lethal dose (LD) of a poison, then one can easily calculate how many atoms or molecules are contained therein (*See* **Table 2-5.**) In scientific notation, 10^{18} is a number representing one billion billions. Thus, cyanide has 4627 billion billions atoms in a lethal dose of 200 mg. This represents a lot of chemical firepower for a just a few cents worth of a substance. In fact, at a cost of $14/lb (454 g) for cyanide, this amount of chemical represents 2270 human lethal doses, or 0.6 cents per lethal dose, or 1.7 lethal doses for a cost of one cent. In reality then, a poison is cheaper than a bullet. A 9-mm round costs approximately 40 cents; for the same price, one can purchase almost 68 lethal doses of cyanide.

2.5. ELEMENTS OF POISONING INVESTIGATIONS

In an attempt to gain some kind of understanding of the type of poisons that have been used in homicidal poisoning cases, the author collected and analyzed 679 cases of known poisonings. The analyses revealed the following information.

Regarding types of poisons used in the homicide, one can see in **Table 2-6** that the top three poisons in order have been: arsenic, cyanide, and strychnine. Regarding the countries in which these poisoning cases occurred, **Table 2-7**, shows their geographic origin. The information might be somewhat biased by the availability of literature in languages other than English. It would be most helpful to have an international clearinghouse for the analysis of criminal cases involving poisons.

2.5.1. Access

We do not know at this point in time which comes first for a poisoner, the knowledge about the poison, or the possession of the poison itself?

Table 2-5
Number of "Killer Molecules" in a Minium Lethal Dose

Poison	Lethal Dose	Gram Molecular Weight	#Molecules
Amatoxin (mushroom)	15 mg	900.00	10×10^{18}
Arsenic	200 mg	74.92	$1,610 \times 10^{18}$
Botulinus toxin	50 ng	150,000	2×10^{11}
Compound"1080"	700 mg	100.03	$4,213 \times 10^{18}$
Cyanide	200 mg	26.02	$4,627 \times 10^{18}$
Strychnine	100 mg	334.45	180×10^{18}
Thallium	1,000 mg	204.37	$2,946 \times 10^{18}$

However, we can hypothesize that more than likely the poisoner seeks out knowledge of a poison that will fulfill the characteristics he or she wishes. Let us assume that the knowledge comes first (*see* **Fig. 2-1**).

2.5.2. Knowledge

Where would one be able to obtain toxicological information? The criminal investigator should consider a number of resources that a poisoner could utilize that would provide valuable information to plan his crime. Among these information resources are the following:

1. Educational background: A poisoner can obtain much information from professional training in biology, chemistry, pharmacology, and/ or medicine.
2. Printed media: The criminal investigator needs to look at the suspect's access to books (both fiction and nonfiction), chemical manuals, magazines, and newspapers for materials relating to poisons or crimes in which poisoning has played a part. Investigators should be especially aware of the availability of "underground" press materials relating to the use of poisons. Protected by the First Amendment to the US Constitution, and supposedly intended for "entertainment purposes," there are currently three such poison references available for easy purchase:

   a. *Assorted Nasties*, by David Harber, Desert Publications, El Dorado, AR, 1993.

Table 2-6
Poison Cases by Poison Used

Poison Used	# Cases	%[a]
Acid	2	0.3%
Acid: boric	1	0.1%
Acid: hydrochloric	1	0.1%
Acid: nitric	1	0.1%
Acid: oxalic	2	0.3%
Acid: sulfuric	3	0.4%
Aconite	5	0.7%
Ammonia	1	0.1%
Ammonium chloride	2	0.3%
Ammonium hydroxide	1	0.1%
Anesthetics	1	0.1%
Antifreeze	1	0.1%
Antimony	9	1.3%
Arsenic	209	30.8%
Atropine	3	0.4%
Bacteria	7	1.0%
Barium acetate	1	0.1%
Belladonna	3	0.4%
Cantharides	1	0.1%
Carburetor cleaner	1	0.1%
Carbon monoxide	7	1.0%
Carcinogen	4	0.4%
Chemicals	1	0.1%
Chloral hydrate	3	0.4%
Chloroform	12	1.8%
Cleaning fluid	1	0.1%
Cocaine	1	0.1%
Copper sulfate	2	0.3%
Corrosives	1	0.1%
Cyanide	61	9.0%
Diazinon	1	0.1%
Drain cleaner	1	0.1%
Drano®	4	0.6%
Drug: antineoplastic	1	0.1%
Drug: antipyrine	1	0.1%
Drug: aspirin	1	0.1%
Drug: barbiturate	4	0.6%
Drug: chlorodyne	2	0.3%
Drug: codeine	1	0.1%
Drug: colchicine	1	0.1%

Table 2-6 continued

Poison Used	# Cases	%[a]
Drug: curacit	1	0.1%
Drug: curare	2	0.3%
Drug: demerol	2	0.3%
Drug: digitalis	4	0.6%
Drug: digoxin	2	0.3%
Drug: innovar	1	0.1%
Drug: insulin	11	1.6%
Drug: laudenum	5	0.7%
Drug: lidocaine	4	0.6%
Drug: morphine	21	3.1%
Drug: navane	1	0.1%
Drug: opiates	3	0.4%
Drug: opium	1	0.1%
Drug: pancuronium	3	0.4%
Drug: paraldehyde	1	0.1%
Drug: pavulon	2	0.3%
Drug: pentothol	1	0.1%
Drug: potassium	3	0.4%
Drug: scopolamine	2	0.3%
Drug: sedatives	1	0.1%
Drug: succinylcholine	3	0.4%
Drug: sucostrin	1	0.1%
Drug: veronal	1	0.1%
Drug: unknown	9	1.3%
Ethanol	1	0.1%
Ether	2	0.3%
Ethylene glycol	1	0.1%
Etorphine	1	0.1%
Fumes/Gas	5	0.7%
Glass	2	0.3%
Hemlock	2	0.3%
Herbicide	1	0.1%
Herbicide: Paraquat	7	1.0%
Herbicide: Pyrilon	1	0.1%
Heroin	2	0.3%
Hyoscine	1	0.1%
Insecticide	1	0.1%
Lead acetate	1	0.1%
Magnesium sulfate	1	0.1%
Mercuric chloride	11	1.6%
Mercury	5	0.7%
Methanol	1	0.1%

Table 2-6 continued

Poison Used	**# Cases**	%[a]
Multiple poisons	14	2.1%
Mushrooms	1	0.1%
Nerve gas: sarin	1	0.1%
Nicotine	1	0.1%
Parathion	1	0.1%
Phencyclidine (PCP)	1	0.1%
Phenol	1	0.1%
Phosphorus	4	0.6%
Plant	1	0.1%
Poison hemlock	1	0.1%
Ratsbane	1	0.1%
Ricin	2	0.3%
Rodenticide	9	1.3%
Selenious acid	1	0.1%
Selenium	1	0.1%
Strychnine	40	5.9%
Thallium	10	1.5%
Unknown: whisky	1	0.1%
Venom	2	0.3%
Warfarin	1	0.1%
Unknown	89	13.1%
TOTAL	679	100.0%

[a] Percentage of total cases.

b. *Silent Death,* by Uncle Fester, Loompanics Unlimited, Port Townsend, WA, 1989, 1997.
c. *The Poisoner's Handbook,* by Maxwell Hutchkinson, Loompanics Unlimited, Port Townsend, WA, 1988.

On the Internet, any individual can be easily led to the availability of these manuals, in which there is an enormous amount of information on poisons, their procurement, production, administration, and lethal dosage, as well as how to avoid detection from the crime. If the criminal investigator finds any of these materials during a search, their suspicions should be aroused immediately.

3. Visual media: In these situations, we have an example of life imitating art. One needs to look for access to movies and television materials relating to poisons or crimes in which poisoning has played a part.
4. Workplace: Labels, manuals, Material Safety Data Sheets (MSDSs), or other materials dealing with chemicals should be investigated.

Table 2-7
Poison Cases by Geographic Location

Country/Location	# Cases	%[a]
Africa	1	0.1%
Africa (South)	13	1.9%
Algeria	1	0.1%
Arctic	1	0.1%
Australia	10	1.5%
Austria	4	0.6%
Belgium	4	0.6%
Canada	6	0.9%
Chile	1	0.1%
China	3	0.4%
Denmark	2	0.3%
France	42	6.2%
Great Britain: England	158	23.3%
Great Britain: N. Ireland	1	0.1%
Great Britain: Scotland	18	2.7%
Great Britain: Wales	2	0.3%
Germany	19	2.8%
Greece	2	0.3%
Guyana	1	0.1%
Hungary	12	1.8%
India	6	0.9%
Ireland	4	0.6%
Israel	1	0.1%
Italy	30	4.4%
Jamaica	1	0.1%
Japan	3	0.4%
Kuwait	1	0.1%
Macedonia	1	0.1%
Mexico	1	0.1%
Netherlands	5	0.7%
New Zealand	2	0.3%
Norway	2	0.3%
Puerto Rico	1	0.1%
Poland	1	0.1%
Russia	5	0.7%
Singapore	1	0.1%
Spain	3	0.4%
St. Helena	1	0.1%
Sweden	1	0.1%
Switzerland	2	0.3%
United States	297	43.7%
Yugoslavia	1	0.1%
?[b]	7	1.0%
TOTAL	679	100.0%

[a]Percentage of total cases.
[b]unknown location

5. Computers: Today, as mentioned, the amount of information that is available to computer users via the Internet or the World Wide Web is incredible. An investigator should consider investigating the possibility of a computer link for information on poisons, or crimes in which poisoning played a part.
6. Word of mouth: Although it is unusual for an offender to talk openly about poisons and their procurement, some cases have relied heavily on the testimony of individuals who have had conversations with the suspect on such matters.

2.5.3. Sources

Once the potential poisoner has the knowledge about the poisonous weapon he has chosen, where does he or she go to obtain the material itself? The criminal investigator should consider some of these sources:

1. Laboratories: Look into the suspect's access to chemical substances that might be found in laboratories in industrial, medical, or educational facilities.
2. Hobbies: Consider chemicals that might be involved in a suspect's hobbies, such as photography, jewelry manufacturing, mineralogy, and so forth.
3. "Underground" catalogues: Believe it or not, there are some individuals who collect poisons, like others collect guns or knives. There is, or was, at least one catalogue available for such individuals, the *JLF* catalogue, based in Indiana. This catalogue of "poisonous non-consumables," which contains a long and detailed disclaimer, allows one to purchase, for example, toxic dried plants, and fungi, and even stated in a recent issue that cobra venom would be "coming soon."
4. Antique drug/chemical bottles: Here is a source of poisons that is often overlooked by investigators. Surprisingly, one can purchase antique chemical bottles with their lethal contents still intact. These items can be obtained from flea markets, Internet auctions, or bottle collectors, and more than likely there is no paper trail of the purchase that leads to the offender.

Selling Antique Chemicals Can Cause Modern Troubles

In order to reduce any potential for unwanted toxicological incidents, the sale and distribution of poisons, legend drugs, and hazardous materials is limited by law to licensed professionals. However, some of these items have found their way into the hands of individuals not licensed to possess or sell such materials. At antique shows and flea markets around the country, and over the computer via Internet auctions, dealers have been found selling antique drug and chemical bottles that still contain toxic contents, including: arsenic, hemlock, mercuric chloride, phenobarbital (a controlled substance), sodium fluoride, and strychnine. How do these individuals come into possession of these drug and chemical containers with hazardous material contents? When queried, most dealers have responded that their sources have been the stocks of old pharmacies and medical offices. They also have stated their belief that the container's contents are now inert due to the extreme age of the product, a belief that, for the most part, is clearly and dangerously erroneous: The compounds of arsenic, for example, are as old as the earth itself, and are as toxic today as when they were first formed millions of years ago.

The Problems These Poisons Present

A poison by any other name is still as dangerous, and the toxicological implications associated with the sale of these hazardous chemicals focus on at least three major problem areas.

Poisons in the Home

The presence of these extremely hazardous substances in the home presents a clear and present danger for accidental and suicidal poisonings. If the collector of antique containers maintains a collection with their contents, then this presents an awesome risk in their home. One case in point involved the son of a pharmacist, who—while in a suicidal frame of mind—packed and swallowed capsules filled with sodium arsenite from his father's collection of antique bottles. The physiological impact of this heavy metal poison almost cost him his life, and the damage to his nervous system was such that even after months of hospitalization and rehabilitation, the arsenic induced peripheral neuropathies could not be totally reversed. The father will probably always regret that this poison was in his home, readily available to his disturbed son.

Poison Procurement with Homicidal or Tampering Intent

It is always of concern to society and to law enforcement personnel that the availability of poisons with a potential for homicidal or tampering use be carefully controlled. Thus, the sale of such substances *must* always be carefully documented in such a manner that proof of transfer of ownership is always maintained. By law, pharmacies are required to maintain a "poison register," to record the sale of any poisonous materials. Selling such poisonous substances without a paper trail could allow homicidal poisoners or tamperers to obtain chemical weapons with no traceable evidence.

Improper Disposal of Extremely Hazardous Substances

In accordance with *Title III* of the *Superfund Amendments Reauthorization Act (SARA)* [P.L. 99-499], it is illegal for any individual or business to dispose of "extremely hazardous substances (EHS)," unless done in a manner consistent with local, state, and federal guidelines. Most knowledgeable businesses wishing to dispose of their hazardous substances will contract with a licensed toxic disposal firm to remove and properly dispose of their unwanted hazardous items. It is also important to note that even if the service of a disposal firm is used for hazardous substances, the original owner is still ultimately responsible for any environmental risk or contamination that may result from the materials. This responsibility cannot be transferred by sale or disposal.

It is important for pharmacists, physicians, and other health professionals to realize that selling their old chemical substances to an individual is not consistent with published guidelines, and that the health professional will ultimately be held legally liable for any toxicological problems that might arise. It is also illegal to dispose of these substances in domestic refuse, or to dump them in such a manner that could lead to contamination of soil or water environments.

The Solution

The solution to keeping such toxic chemicals out of the hands of the lay public is quite simple. Antique bottles containing hazardous contents must never be sold. The hazardous contents must be carefully removed and disposed of in a manner that is consistent with local, state, and federal legal guidelines. Detailed records must be maintained that document proper disposal of any hazardous chemical substance. Health and law enforcement professionals must remain vigilant regarding the sale of these chemicals to unlicensed individuals, and must clearly and emphatically state to the sellers the dangers of this practice. Any seller who refuses to withdraw these materials from sale should be immediately reported to the local office of the Food and Drug Administration (FDA), Consumer Products Safety

Commission (CPSC), and the Environmental Protection Agency (EPA).

Once the poisoner has both knowledge and weapon, the next step is to deliver the weapon to the intended victim, and carry out the crime. We must now look at the poisoner himself, to attempt to gain some understanding of what makes this type of individual tick.

2.6. REFERENCES

Deichman WB, Henschler D, Keil G: What is there that is not poison? A study of the *Third Defense* by Paracelsus. *Arch Toxicol,* 1986; 58:207–213.

Thompson CJS: *Poison Mysteries in History, Romance and Crime,* J.B. Lippincott, Philadelphia, 1924.

2.7. SUGGESTED READINGS

Ellenhorn MJ: Ellenhorn's *Medical Toxicology: Diagnosis and Treatment of Human Poisoning,* 2nd ed. Williams & Wilkins, Baltimore, MD, 1997.

Farrell M: *Poisons and Poisoners: An Encyclopedia of Homicidal Poisonings.* Robert Hale, London, 1992.

Ferner RF: *Forensic Pharmacology: Medicines, Mayhem, and Malpractice.* Oxford University Press, New York, NY, 1996.

Goldfrank LR, Flomenbaum NE, Lewin NA, etal. Goldfrank's *Toxicologic Emergencies,* 6th ed. Appleton & Lange, Stamford, CT, 1998.

Haddad LM, Shannon MW, Winchester JF: *Clinical Management of Poisoning and Drug Overdose,* 3rd ed. W.B. Saunders, Philadelphia, PA, 1998.

Chapter 3

POISONERS

> *"When you consider what a chance women have to poison their husbands, it's a wonder there isn't more of it done."* —Kim Hubbard

As stated in the introduction to this work, the poisoner has remained shrouded in mystery for centuries. Let us now examine what we know about the poisoner as an offender, and what we think we know about the poisoner.

3.1. TYPES

One way to look at the motivation of a poisoner is to study how the victim is selected: does the poisoner target a specific individual, or has he chosen a target at random? The motives of these two groups of poisoners are very different.

The following method of classification of poisoners based on victim specificity and degree of planning involved was developed by the author. There are two major groups, relating to targeting or choosing a victim. Each group has two sub-groups, relating to the speed with which the crime is planned and then carried out.

3.1.1. *Type S (where a* specific *victim is targeted)*

Motives for this group of poisoners include: money, elimination, jealousy, revenge, or political ambition.

Sub-Group S
(a poisoning *slowly* planned, with a carefully selected poison)

An example of this type of poisoner would be a woman, angry with her husband, who goes to the library, reads about a particular poison, procures the chemical, and decides the best manner of administration to the victim. Type S/S = Specific/Slow.

Sub-Group Q (a poisoning *quickly* planned)

The crime in this sub-group is a spontaneous decision, with a poison selected as a weapon of opportunity. An example of this type of poisoner would be a woman who is angry with her husband, and quickly takes a can of herbicide from storage and adds some to his food while preparing a meal. Type S/Q = Specific/Quick.

3.1.2. *Type R (where a* random *victim is targeted)*

Motives for this group of poisoners include: ego, tampering, boredom, or sadism.

Sub-Group S
(a poisoning *slowly* planned with a carefully selected poison)

An example of this type of poisoner would be a tamperer intent on industrial blackmail, who adulterates a food/drug with a carefully selected poisonous substance. This group would also include terrorists. Type R/S = Random/Slow.

Sub-Group Q (a poisoning *quickly* planned)

The crime in this case is spontaneously committed, with a poison selected as a weapon of opportunity. An example of this type of poisoner would be an employee who—upset with his employer—quickly picks up a toxic substance and adulterates a batch of a consumer product (food, drug, cosmetic, etc.) to which he/she has access. Type R/Q = Random/Quick.

Whenever we think we have been able to classify poisoners, we must remember to be aware of the "camouflaged" poisoner! In this situation, a poisoner gives the appearance of being a Type R, but is in reality a Type S. An example of this type of poisoner would be an offender who poisons his spouse by tampering with her medication, then places similar tampered containers in a retail store to make the death of the victim appear to be random. There are various recorded cases of this type of poisoner at work. Among the more infamous cases, listed chronologically, are:

- Christiana Edmunds (Brighton, UK, 1871): Poisoned chocolates in a confectioner's shop with strychnine, and one innocent child became a random victim. Her specific target was the wife of the man who thwarted her affection.
- Ronald Clark O'Bryan (Pasadena, Texas, 1974): Poisoned Halloween candy of neighborhood children with cyanide. His son, whom he killed to collect a life insurance premium, was the specific victim. He was also convicted of three attempts on the other neighborhood children, which he had planned in order to make the crime appear like the actions of a deranged tamperer.
- Stella Maudine Nickell (Auburn, Washington, 1986): Poisoned Excedrin® capsules with cyanide to cover up the specific murder of her husband for insurance money. One random victim died, making the crime appear to be the work of a tamperer.
- Joseph Meling (Tumwater, Washington, 1991): Poisoned Sudafed 12-Hour® capsules with cyanide, to cover up the specific murder attempt on his wife. One random victim died, also making the crime appear to be the work of a tamperer.
- Paul Agutter (Athelstaneford, Scotland, 1994): Poisoned tonic water with atropine, to cover up the specific murder attempt on his wife. Eight victims suffered from his atropine tampering intoxication, but there were no deaths in this case.

Investigators should remember from these cases always to question whether product tampering might actually be an attempt to cover up a specific homicide by throwing their investigation off the correct track.

This classification system has been summarized in **Fig. 3-1**.

3.2. MISCONCEPTIONS ABOUT POISONERS

It is important to correct some common poison and poisoner myths that exist in the minds of the general population. Among these myths

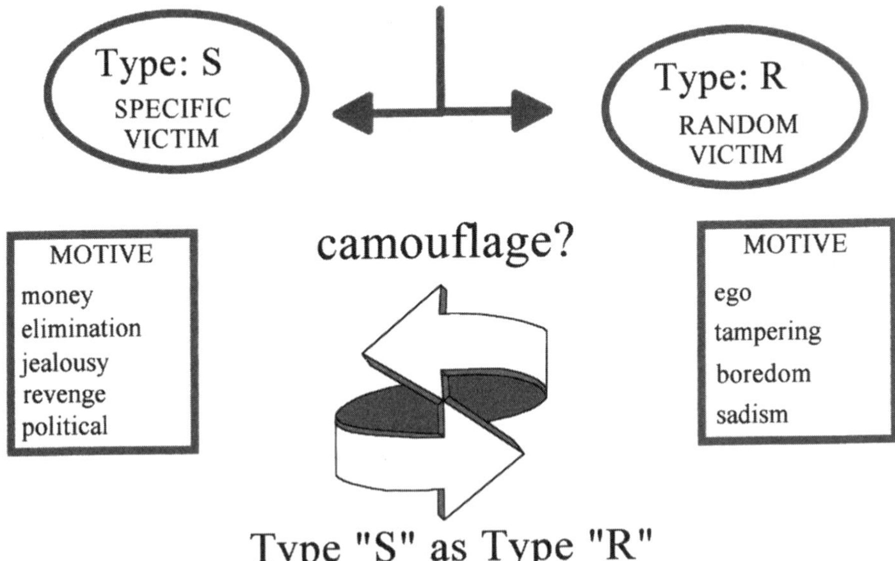

is that most poisoners are female. In actuality, the majority of poisoners that have been detected have been male. (The words "have been detected" are very important.) This could lead one to speculation that females are more successful escaping detection.

Poison could be the favorite weapon of the female murderer, however. An analysis of the 49 women executed for murder in Great Britain in a 48-year period (1843–1890) showed that regarding motive, 22 (45%) were motivated by money, 10 (20%) were motivated by sexual triangles, and in 17 (35%) of the cases the motive was unclear. Regarding their weapon, 29 (59%) of the women used poison, with arsenic having been used by 23 (79%) of these female poisoners.

Another common myth is that for every poison, there is an emergency antidote. (It should also be emphasized here that the proper word for this type of drug is "antidote" not "anecdote," which is sometimes used erroneously.) In reality, there are currently only five (FDA) approved drugs that can make a life-and-death difference in the poisoning emergency. These antidotes are listed in **Table 3-1**.

The last myth, and a question very commonly asked is: Does a perfect undetectable poison exist? The answer to this question could be a yes or no, depending on how we describe the word "undetect-

Table 3-1
Critical Medical Antidotes

Poison used against	Antidote
Organophosphates: nerve gases, insecticides	Atropine
Cyanide	Cyanide Antidote Package® (Lilly)
Allergic shock	Epinephrine
Opiates, narcotics	Naloxone
Carbon monoxide	Oxygen

able." The answer should be "no," if we consider that, if there was such an undetectable substance, how would we ever know it existed? If it has a name, someone must have detected it at least once to name it, and therefore anything with a name is theoretically detectable. However, the answer could be "yes," if we mean by "undetectable" that the chance it will be routinely seen in a toxicological analysis is slim. If poisoning is suspected, and the analytical experts are given proper guidelines, almost every toxic chemical can be identified. However, if there are no guidelines to assist them, it is rather like looking for a molecular needle in a chemical haystack. If the substance is not one screened for in their normal substance panels, it will very likely go undetected. The problem is not the perfection of the poison, but the imperfection of the analytical process. Here it should also be emphasized that a "negative" toxicological screen does not mean that there is no poison in the specimen, but rather that all the poisons routinely tested for in the analysis are absent. There could be other, more exotic, poisonous compounds that remain undetected.

3.3. POISONER SCHEMATIC

In order for law enforcement to stand a better chance of solving poisoning homicides, it is important to understand why an individual would choose this type of weapon over more traditional weapons like a gun, knife, club, or rope. In order to answer this question, and to develop a Criminal Investigative Analysis (sometimes referred to as a "psychological profile") of this type of offender, the criminal investigation community must carry out a carefully planned study of convicted poisoners, to look for commonalities in their background and behavior. Such a study would be of immense value in guiding the homicide investigator in his awesome task. Currently, the plans to carry out this critical research are in the early design stages.

However, we can make some hypotheses about this type of individual by looking at the personalities involved with the published cases of poisonings in which there have been convictions. Some things are common with these types of poisoning offenders. Poisoners are for the most part: cunning, avaricious, cowardly (physically or mentally nonconfrontational), child-like in their fantasy, and somewhat artistic (meaning they can design the plan for the murder in as much detail as if they were writing the script for a play).

Why does the poison murderer select this weapon as the means of getting to the goal? One of the major reasons is that they stand a very good chance of getting away with the crime. Other reasons include the fact that a poison allows completion of the assault without physical confrontation with the victim. The poisoner is truly an intelligent-coward, or we could say has the mind set of an "enfant-terrible" (incorrigible child) in the body of an adult. This is a very dangerous combination. If one also looks at many, if not most, of the male poisoners who have been tried and convicted, one will see that they tend to deal with conflict in a manner that is not physically confrontational. These characteristics have been summarized in **Fig. 3-2.**

3.4. POISONER THOUGHT PROCESS

What goes through the poisoner's mind as they are planning their crime? Certainly all behavior is caused. The instigating force is the *motive*, or the force that moves them to the decision to eliminate that individual that stands between themselves and their goal. First they say "I want to do something," and that is the motive to their crime. Their *intent* is to remove the obstacle that stands between them and their goal. Next they have to have the *means*, which indicates that they have access to both the knowledge of the poison and the poison itself. They also have to have the *opportunity*, which means by having knowledge of the victim's habits, they have access to their intended target. And lastly, they are concerned with the detection of their crime. They try to ensure that they have no witnesses to all the crime aspects,

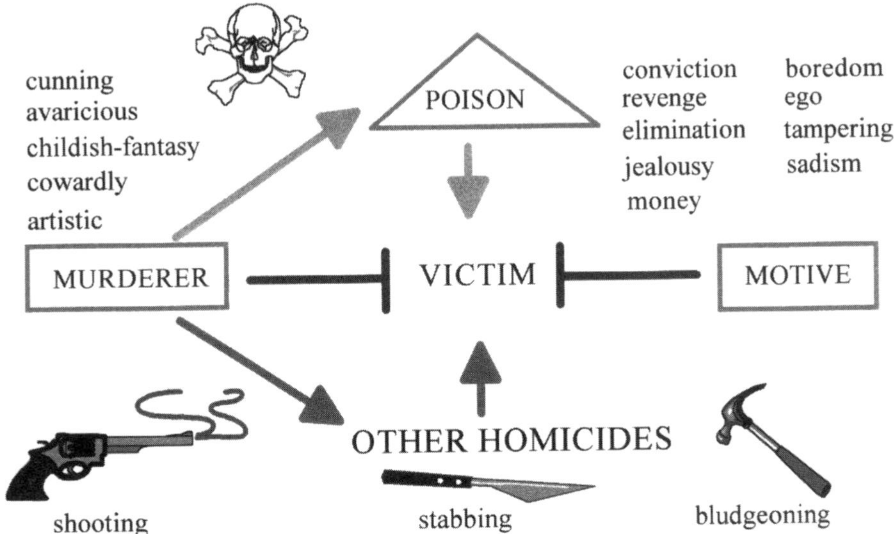

have enough distance from the crime, leave no visible signs of the crime, and believe they can escape detection. These thought processes are summarized in **Fig. 3-3**.

3.5. PSYCHOLOGICAL PROFILE OF POISONERS

In the personality of the poisoner, the investigator will probably find some of the following traits: an absolute defiance of legal authority; a refusal to accept any moral basis for life; killing in order to gain either emotionally or materially; an unfortunate married life for the offender; a childhood in which the poisoner has been either spoiled by parents or reared in an unhappy home; a tendency to turn the victim into an object with no feelings; an abnormal life with wife, children, or home; feeling they have failed to make any kind of impression on life; a tendency to be daydreamers and fantasists; a touch of an artistic temperament; possible connections with the medical world as physicians, nurses, pharmacists, dentists, other health care workers, or laboratory workers familiar with chemicals; possession of vanity in thinking they cannot be discovered, in that they carefully calculate the odds and believe they can get away with the crime; a limited mind without sympathy; and weak, cowardly, and avaricious temperment (Glaister, 1954; Rowland, 1960).

One sees in the childish personality of the poisoner an immature desire for their own way, and a dreamy, romantic disposition. There seems to

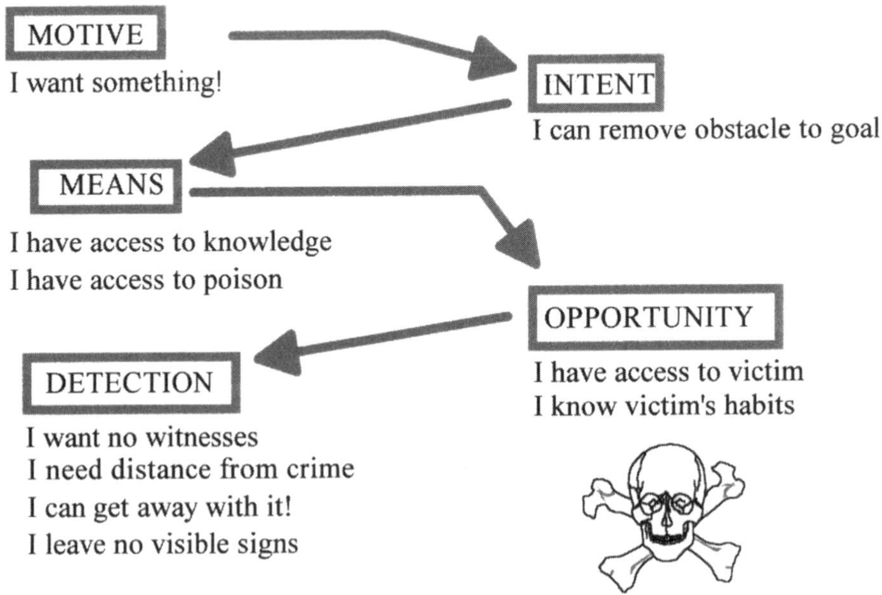

be something in the poisoners that keeps them permanently immature; they never seem to grow up. They try to make the world obey their will by cheating it in minor ways, and thereby stealing what it refuses to give them.

As far as the poisoners' motives for murder, they are not much different from other homicides, in that they usually revolve around money (insurance); elimination of goal-blocker; jealousy ("lover's triangle"); revenge (make them pay); sadism (make them suffer); conviction (political motives, e.g. assassination, terrorism); boredom (wants to have fun by having a challenge of wits with law enforcement); and ego (belief in mental superiority).

3.6. PUBLIC PERCEPTION OF POISONERS

When one looks at how the general public views the poisoner, one can often see a sort of morbid fascination with this type of crime. However, in general, the public have a special hatred for the poisoner's sinister nature. The public generally believes that poison is a coward's weapon, because it is administered unemotionally and by stealth, often gradually over a long period of time. The administration of the poison is done in full recognition of the victim's often prolonged suffering. The public reviles the poisoner for his lack of pity.

3.7. THE TOXICOMANIAC

A very rare mental condition is the "Toxicomaniac," or lover of poisons. They relish the feeling of power provided to them by their weapon. The major example of this rather rare condition is the English case of Graham Frederick Young, who from the age of 11 became obsessed with poisons, and eventually caused several deaths and many ill effects by experimenting on his relatives and coworkers with poison. He treated the victims not as humans, but as if they were rats in a toxicological study. His story was told in the black comedy 1995 British film, "The Young Poisoner's Handbook,"although most homicide investigators should fail to see humor in the film.

3.8. STATISTICAL ANALYSIS OF HOMICIDAL POISONINGS

In an attempt to shed some light on the poisoner, the author collected and analyzed 679 documented poisoning crimes. What follows is the results of these analyses.

3.8.1. Most Common Poison Used

As can be seen in **Table 3-2**, the most commonly used poisons in order have been the "Big Three" consisting of arsenic, cyanide, and strychnine, along with morphine and chloroform. These three poisons were involved in 46% of all the poisoning cases analyzed.

3.8.2. Poisoner's Background

This analysis indicated that the majority (71%) came from what could be called the general public; that is private citizens. These results can be seen in **Table 3-3**.

3.8.3. Poisoner's Gender

This analysis produced the result that the majority of the offenders were male (46%); females represented 39% of the cases. This analysis must be

Table 3-2
Most Common Poisons Used

Poison	#	%
Arsenic	209	31%
Cyanide	61	9%
Strychnine	40	6%
Morphine	21	3%
Chloroform	12	2%
Total	343	50%

[a](*n* = 679)

Table 3-3
Poisoner's Background

Group	#	%
Public	479	71%
Physician	52	8%
Political	29	4%
Nurse	24	4%
Other	33	5%
Unknown	62	9%
Total	679	100%

[a](*n* = 679)

looked at with the caveat that in 16% of the cases, the gender of the offender was unknown, as well as the fact that these cases only represent incidents that were detected. It could be once again that females were more successful at remaining undetected in the crime. (*See* **Table 3-4.**)

3.8.4. Number of Victims

In 33% of the cases, there had been multiple victims, which were divided into separate incidents. This would indicate that in almost one-third of these the poisoner was a serial killer. (*See* **Table 3-5.**)

3.8.5. Poisoner's Motive

In looking at the recorded motives for the crime, it usually involved love or money. (*See* **Table 3-6.**)

3.8.6. Offender's Conviction Status

In 96% of the cases, the suspect was convicted of the crime. Many of the remaining cases were dismissed under a cloud of suspicion, but

Table 3-4
Poisoner's Gender

Gender	#	%
Male	311	46%
Female	260	39%
Unknown	108	16%
Total	679	100%

[a] (n = 679)

Table 3-5
Number of Victims

Known victims	#	%
Single	443	66%
Multiple	236	35%
Unknown	0	0%
Total	679	100%

[a](n = 679)

prosecutors were unable to prove the case beyond a reasonable doubt. (*See* **Table 3-7**).

3.8.7. Multiple Offenders on Victim(s)

In 90% of the cases, only a single offender was involved in the crime. Multiple offender cases, although rare, are usually easier to convict, because there is the possibility of the two participants providing evidence against each other. (*See* **Table 3-8**).

3.8.8. Gender of the Offender vs Number of Victims

It has been speculated by some that if the female is less easily detected in her crime, she has a greater opportunity to carry out her deeds on multiple victims, over a longer period of time. In an analysis of an enhanced 769 cases collected by the author, it was found that when one looks at gender vs number of victims, in the cases involving a female offender, 41% of them had multiple victims; for males it was 34%. This would seem to indicate that there is some greater chance of

Table 3-6
Poisoner's Motive

Motive	#	%
Insurance (individual)	176	26%
Domestic	58	9%
Political extremism	47	7%
Personal cause	76	11%
Other	129	19%
Unknown	193	29%

[a]($n = 679$)

Table 3-7
Offender's Conviction Status

Status	#	%
Convicted	647	96%
Acquitted	32	5%
Unknown	0	0%
Total	679	100%

[a]($n = 679$)

Table 3-8
Multiple Offenders on Victim(s)

Offenders	#	%
Single	606	90%
Multiple	73	11%
Unknown	0	0%
Total	679	100%

[a]($n = 679$)

Table 3-9
Offender Gender vs Number of Victims

Offender gender	Single victim	%	Multiple victims	%	Total	%
Female	170	59%	118	41%	288	37%
Male	229	66%	117	34%	346	45%
Unknown	114	84%	21	16%	135	18%
Total	513	68%	256	33%	769	100%

[a](n) = 769

females having multiple victims, but it might not be a significant difference between the genders. (*See* **Table 3-9**.)

As can be seen from this chapter's discussion of the poisoner, there is much more that we need to determine about this type of criminal offender. To be able to lift the veil of secrecy that surrounds them, it will take a concentrated and coordinated effort on an international scale to look at commonalities and possible cultural differences on the use of poison as a weapon for murder.

3.9. REFERENCES

Glaister J: *The Power of Poison*. William Morrow, New York, NY, 1954, pp. 153–182.
Rowland J: *Poisoner in the Dock*. Arco Publications, London, 1960, pp. 230–237.

3.10. SUGGESTED READING

Kelleher MD, Kelleher CL: *Murder Most Rare: The Female Serial Killer*. Praeger, Westport, CT, 1998.
Pollack O: *The Criminality of Women*. Greenwood Press Publishers, Westport, CT, 1978.
Sparrow G: *Women Who Murder: Crimes and the Feminine Logic Behind Them*. Abelard-Schuman, New York, NY, 1970.
Thorwald J: *Proof of Poison*. Thames and Hudson, London, 1966.

Chapter 4

VICTIMS

> *"Most signs and symptoms associated with natural disease can be produced by some poison, and practically every sign and symptom observed in poisoning can be mimicked by those associated with natural diseases."*
> —L. Adelson

Most often the victim of poisoning will appear rather natural in death. In effect, poisoning is murder in slow motion, as it may take a long period of time, depending on the dose and the poison that has been selected as the weapon. Two major factors that determine lethality of a substance are (1) concentration and (2) duration of exposure.

4.1. WHO GETS POISONED?

Poisoning murders can be classified into a number of groupings depending on the motive for homicide.

There can be a suicidally motivated parent, who wants to take the children with them. A good example of this type of killing would be use of cyanide by Joseph Goebbels and his wife in 1945 to murder their children in Hitler's Berlin bunker as the Allied troops approached and the end of the Third Reich was near.

Another type of poisoning death can be due to an unintentional homicidal poisoning (manslaughter), which might result from an accidental drug overdose, as in the death of comedian John Belushi.

Another interesting incident was the 1954 British case of Arthur Ford, who in his wish to sexually arouse two of his female office coworkers, accidentally killed them with his use of Cantharides ("Spanish Fly").

A death may also result from administration of a harmful substance in an attempt to induce behavior modification in a child in order to stop what is deemed improper behavior (e.g., bed wetting, nail biting, not following parental instructions, etc.). Several deaths have been documented from the administration of powdered black pepper (*Piper negrum*), which resulted in an aspiration death of the child.

One of the more recently discussed abnormal psychological conditions is what has become known as "Munchausen Syndrome by Proxy." This condition was named after the famous German storyteller Baron von Munchausen, who was a famous teller of fabulously unbelievable tales. This syndrome is a phenomenon in which a mentally ill parent administers poison to the child in order to draw attention to themselves. They enjoy being the center of attention, and by using a child as the object of the medical emergency, they in effect become the center of this attention by proxy. The offender gets some personal psychological reward from having doctors listen and begins to exaggerate the symptoms. This type of poisoner is usually a mother, who may show many of the following characteristics:

1. Comes from a background where she was ignored and unrecognized;
2. Has a history of being abused herself;
3. May consider the relationship she had with her obstetrician the most intense, personal, and rewarding she had ever had; and is attempting to transfer this role to the child's pediatrician;
4. Many have some nursing training; and
5. May have a history of weaving false tales of medical problems. This type of poisoning event is considered a form of child abuse. In most cases, the father is usually oblivious to the activities, or may be in subconscious collusion with the perpetrator.

The timely issue of euthanasia of the elderly and terminally ill by homicidal poisoning, in private homes as well as in nursing homes, has come to national attention in the past few years. Dr. Jack Kevorkian's process of right to die has brought this type of poisoning to the forefront of nightly news around the country. Its popularity is also evidenced by the euthanasia guidebook *Final Exit*, and the existence of the "Hemlock Society," which provides instructions to those wishing to end their own lives because of terminal illness.

The emphasis of this investigative work concentrates mainly on intentional homicidal poisoning, which is always considered first degree murder because of the element of premeditation.

4.2. INVESTIGATIVE CONSIDERATIONS

What indices might the homicide investigator utilize to help him or her determine that a poisoning murder may have occurred? Investigators should look for friends/relatives arousing suspicion, as well as suspicious circumstances that surround the death. Some indicators might include: the sudden death of the victim after eating, drinking, or going into the bathroom, or if poison containers were found near the deceased. In a suicide, the latter might well be the case, although it could be a murder masquerading as a suicide.

The antemortem (before death) clinical course might indicate that the deceased exhibited symptoms consistent with a poisoning, but it is easy for an investigator to be misled. One would think that an autopsy of the body would clearly reveal that the cause of death was other than natural. However, research conducted in 1958 indicated that 10% of homicides are not detected. It is alarming that when autopsy results were compared to death certificates, an error rate of approximately 50% was found in the cause of death as indicated on the certificates.

4.3. DISTINCTIVE PATHOLOGICAL FINDINGS

- Does the victim exhibit no morphological changes that can be attributed to direct chemical action by a toxic agent? Poisonous substances that might be considered in such cases include the following: acute CNS depressants (alcohols, ethers, sedatives, chloroform, hypnotics, and so forth); chemical asphyxiant gases (carbon monoxide, hydrogen cyanide); organo-phosphate insecticides (OPI; malathion or parathion); and alkaloidal compounds (strychnine, opiates).
- Are systemic lesions present without obvious injury at the site of entry? Poisonous substances that might be considered include arsine or nitrobenzene.
- Is an injury present at site of entry that does not exhibit remote or systemic evidence of direct cell damage? Poisonous substances that

might be considered include substances that cause immediate cellular necrosis (corrosives) or gaseous irritants (chlorine, sulfur dioxide).

- Are local and systemic injuries present? Poisonous substances that might be considered include heavy metals such as mercuric chloride, arsenic, antimony, lead, and so forth.

4.4. CLASSIC SYMPTOMS OF POISONING

To follow are some visible clues that should alert criminal investigators and health care workers that a victim may have been poisoned:

1. Hair loss: often found with chronic intoxication from the heavy metals (e.g., arsenic, antimony, thallium). It is surprising how often this clue is overlooked.
2. Fever: results from the activation of body's defense systems.
3. Constricted pupils ("miosis"): often found from opiate compounds (morphine, codeine, heroin, etc.) and organophosphate insecticides (OPI) and so forth.
4. Dilated pupils ("mydriasis"): can be found with the Solanaceous plant alkaloids, such as atropine, scopolamine, and hyoscyamine, as well as insulin, cocaine, nicotine, and so forth.
5. Odor: some poisons have characteristic odors that may be detectable on the victim (arsenic = garlic, vacor = peanuts, nitrobenzene = shoe polish, and so on).
6. Oral burns: the mouth area or face may exhibit burns caused by caustics and corrosives compounds (acids and alkalais, e.g., sodium hydroxide [lye]).
7. Gastrointestinal effects (diarrhea): may be caused by many poisons, especially the heavy metals.
8. Skin color: cherry-red color results from carbon monoxide, blue color (cyanosis) from nitrites (methemoglobinemia).
9. Vomiting: results from stomach irritation (arsenic, antimony, aconite, acids, alkalais, colchicine, cantharides, phosphorus, mercury, iodine, etc.).
10. Injection tracks: from multiple administrations of poisons by the parenteral route.
11. Skin speckling (which looks like raindrops hitting the surface of a dusty road): can be caused by chronic doses of arsenic.
12. Stomach cramps: a classic sign of chronic poisoning.

Table 4-1
Some Common Poisons and Their Symptoms

Symptom	Poison
Hair loss	Thallium, other heavy metals
Fever	Multiple poisons
Constricted pupils (miosis)	Opiates, organophosphate pesticides
Dilated pupils (mydriasis)	Alkaloids, insulin
Garlic odor	Arsenic, antimony, etc.
Peanut odor	Vacor (rodenticide)
Bitter almonds odor	Cyanide
Shoe polish odor	Nitrobenzene
Oral burns	Corrosives (lye, acids)
Diarrhea	Heavy metals
Cherry red skin color	Carbon monoxide
Blue skin color (cyanosis)	Nitrites
Vomiting	Multiple irritant poisons
Injection tracts	Insulin, drugs of abuse
Skin speckling	Arsenic (chronic)
Stomach cramps	Multiple poisons
Nail changes ("Mees' lines," brittle)	Heavy metals (arsenic)
Convulsions	Strychnine, cocaine, pesticides
Coma	Depressants, hypnotics
Paralysis	Botulism, heavy metals
Abrupt onset of symptoms	Multiple poisons

13. Brittle nails and "Mees' lines" (white lines across the nail beds): heavy metals can change the nail structure.
14. Convulsions: caused by strychnine, organo-phosphate compounds, camphor, cyanide, and so forth.
15. Coma: caused by opiates, hypnotics, sedatives, carbon monoxide (CO), carbon dioxide (CO_2), ethanol, phenols, and so forth.
16. Paralysis (general or partial): owing to nerve system alterations caused by botulism, cyanide, thallium, arsenic, and so forth.
17. Abrupt onset of symptoms: sudden appearance of symptoms in a previously healthy individual. This is summarized for the investigator in **Table 4-1.**

With the correct determination that the victim has been the target of a poisoner's efforts, the focus turns to the crime scene. The role of the investigator is then to gather evidence that will eventually lead to the source of the poison, and the poisoner him or herself.

4.5. REFERENCES

Adelson L: *Pathology of Homicide*, Charles C. Thomas, Springfield, IL, 1974.

Dreisbach RH, Robertson WO: *Handbook of Poisoning*, 12th ed. Appleton & Lange, Norwalk, CT, 1987.

4.6. SUGGESTED READINGS

Ferner RE: *Forensic Pharmacology: Medicines, Mayhem, and Malpractice*. Oxford University Press, New York, NY, 1996.

Chapter 5

Crime Scene Investigation

> *"Murder is first conceived in the heart. But if it remains there—as it often does—it is no crime, though it may well be a sin. It is the acceptance of the idea of murder as a possible means of getting what one wants that is the decisive step. For most normal and sane people the idea is still-born. They smile to themselves and say 'What am I thinking of?' The thought passes, and is lost in the limbo of forgotten fantasy. But if the thought is not forgotten? If it recurs? If it is first half-accepted and then embraced? From this point we have a woman who intends to murder and we pass to the field of strategy and tactics."*—Gerald Sparrow

The prime directive for gathering evidence of poisoning at a death scene is to remember the proper "chain of custody." Nothing can break a case assumed to be solid more easily than the defense being able to prove reasonable possibility that evidence could have been tampered with before the trial.

The object that initiated the investigation was the victim, and so it is with the victim that we begin search for answers to important questions. What has become known as "victimology" is a study of the victim that will hopefully reveal clues that can answer questions of *why* and *who*. Why was the person possibly a target? By answering this question, one begins to determine if there was any individual who would have anything to gain either physically or mentally from the victim's death. One needs to get a complete history of the victim, including a detailed financial background.

Remember that the victim him or herself is the most important crime scene.

Regarding the crime scene, with poisoning there can be multiple locations that came into play during planning and carrying out murder. Each location can yield important clues that must be included in the complete case investigation. Some of the locations and the clues that are important are as follows:

1. Where the victim was *found* (vomited material, clothes containing poison residue);
2. Where the poison was *administered* (medicine bottles, food/beverage containers);
3. Where the poison was *disposed* of (storage areas, trash containers, sink traps);
4. Where the poison was *prepared* (poison residues on tools, utensils, clothes, containers); and
5. Where the poison was *procured* (stolen items being looked for, receipts of purchase, signing of a poison register).

The criminal investigator needs to closely look at the environment of the crime scene, regarding place and time. Does the crime scene show that it might have been manipulated, in other words, is it too clean?

How many offenders might have been involved with this crime? With poisonings, the vast majority will involve a single offender on a single victim. This type of crime is not a group activity, although a few cases have been documented in which multiple offenders have poisoned a victim or victims.

5.1. PHYSICAL EVIDENCE

The analysis of whether a crime scene appears organized or disorganized can often yield valuable information on the mind set of the killer. The poisoner will usually exhibit some characteristics of both the organized and disorganized personality. Some of the organized characteristics include:

1. A planned offense, and
2. Weapon/evidence often absent from the crime scene.

Among the characteristics left at the crime scene by the disorganized individual one may find:

1. The victim location is known;
2. The body is left in plain view; and
3. The body is left at the death scene.

The criminal investigator needs to look carefully at the death scene to answer some of the following important questions: Does the body disposition show the possibility of an unnatural death? Are there items intentionally left, or strangely missing from the scene?

Are there any unusual odors at the death scene? Remember to watch out for the masking effect of tobacco smoke on unusual odors associated with some poisons (e.g. cyanide, solvents, fumes). It is best that there be no smoking at the crime scene.

Is there evidence of "staging" (purposeful alteration of the crime scene)? Remember that with the poisoner, the scene will be mostly left in a natural state, except that the vehicle for administering the poison may have been removed or cleaned.

5.2. INVESTIGATIVE CONSIDERATIONS

If there was one, interview the first aid responder as to what the victim looked like before therapy was attempted. Was the victim cleaned up? If so, where are the materials that were used in the cleaning, as they may contain valuable toxicological evidence.

5.3. SEARCH WARRANTS

If the poisoner does not think he will be suspected, the area of preparation may not be cleaned up, as it is the "den of security." Why hide something you don't think an investigator will ever look for? It is important for investigators to stay within the "four corners" of the warrant. On the warrant, specify exact location and items that need to be investigated. Of course, in order to obtain a warrant, there must be "probable cause," as defined under the Fourth Amendment to the US Constitution. Above all, remember that a poison could be found anywhere, and one must look into such areas as wastebaskets, sink traps, garbage, and work locations. The poison most likely will be in small quantities (<200 g), and will not be a 50-lb barrel glowing with some strange iridescent color in the corner of the home.

There are related items to search for, and the criminal investigator should consider all of the following: publications on poisons, receipts for procurement of chemicals, medical publications, poison recipe cards, chemical catalogues, diaries/journals, and evidence that may be contained in computer files and records.

Other points to be considered when executing a search warrant include some of the following: Read over the search warrant and affidavit prior to execution of the warrant, and become very familiar with all details of the proposed search. Remember to leave a copy of the search warrant at each location that has been searched. Leave a receipt, and note the date/time of execution and securing of evidence. Maintain a complete and detailed inventory of seized properties. Do not consume any edible materials at the site, because one never knows if evidence has been destroyed, or in the case of a poisoner, whether edibles are tainted.

5.4. POISONING DEATHS COMPARED WITH OTHER TYPES OF VIOLENT DEATHS

As a crime, poisoning exhibits some nuances usually different from the more violent and traumatic homicides. The offender is usually secretive, quiet, and covert, and will not confide in others about the intention or execution of the murder. The victim will usually exhibit no external signs of violence. The crime almost always involves careful planning and cool deliberation (the murderer engineers the well-conceived opportunity). The offender is most thoughtfully and seriously concerned with preventing discovery of the crime, and the poisoner is probably the most cunning of murderers. The offender usually possesses a high degree of skill and knowledge of the victim's routine/personal habits, and will usually act alone; thus, there will be an absence of witnesses. The offender kills because he really believes he can kill and get away with the crime. A poisoning murder is usually an intimate or "household" crime, with the principals usually united by close emotional ties (the marital bond is most common).

Additional contrasts are that the victim of a poisoning is defenseless, with no protection, and therefore will not likely exhibit any defensive kind of evidence. The offender has a high degree of knowledge of the lethal potentialities of the poison used, as he has more than likely thoroughly researched the poison.

It has been stated that poisoning is the least used method of homicide, accounting for 3–6% of known homicide cases. With all the difficulties involved in a poisoning homicide, it is one of the most difficult homicides to prove. Homicidal poisoning is almost always murder, never manslaughter (unless the offender is judged to be legally insane), because of the premeditation, deliberation, and intent to kill.

5.5. INVESTIGATING A CRIMINAL POISONING

In order to better the chances of detecting the murder by poison, all death investigations should be handled as homicide cases until the facts prove otherwise.

To begin an investigation, it is necessary to gather some facts that may help determine if the death might have been due to a poisoning incident. If the victim is still alive, ask questions that deal with symptoms, how he/she feels, and if these symptoms' onset coincided with a common event. If the victim is dead, ask these same questions of any other individuals that had contact with the deceased. (Always remember, you may be interviewing the poisoner himself). Essential information that needs to be gathered has been summarized in **Table 5-1.**

If the criminal investigator determines that a poison is likely to have been involved in the death, then he/she must determine the possible source of the poisonous weapon. It is imperative to look for a possible paper trail that might show taking possession. If the poison was procured at a pharmacy, ask to see the pharmacy's "Poison Register," which should indicate date, purchaser's name and address, name of the substance, amount purchased, and intended use. Was there a commercial source, such as a chemical supply company, that might have purchasing records? Is there a possible computer trail that shows purchase of the material over the Internet? Did the offender have any connection with an industrial or educational institution that would have allowed him to steal the material?

5.6. PHYSICAL EVIDENCE

The criminal investigator should take into evidence any and all of the following types of materials: remains of food and drink, drugs, medicines, chemicals in the home, glasses, bottles, spoons, syringes, and soiled linen or clothing.

Table 5-1
Information to Obtain During a Poisoning Investigation

What was the location of victim when symptoms first appeared?
What were the symptoms?
Did someone give the poison intentionally? (Who might have done it, what was the motive?)
Did the victim administer the poison him/herself (accidental or intentional); if so, why?
Who called for help (when and how)?
What did the victim do just prior to appearance of symptoms?
What did the victim eat or drink prior to symptoms?
Did the victim abuse any drugs or controlled substances (which could have been adulterated)?
Was food or medication requested or offered? (Who prepared it, and who served it?)
Did any other person consume the same items, and if so, how are they?
Was the victim in the habit of consuming the substance in question?
Was the victim in the habit of consuming any type of alcohol not intended for drinking?
Did the victim eat or drink anything after the symptoms first appeared?
Did the victim take any medicine before the appearance of the symptoms?
What was the victim's general health condition?
Was the victim recently unhappy, depressed, jealous, or angry?
Did the victim have money on his/her person prior to the symptoms?
What was the condition of his estate, and did he/she owe large sums of money?
Who would inherit the victim's estate, and do they have immediate financial needs?
Did the victim have any recent difficulties with his employment?
Was anyone jealous of the victim because of his position (who might be promoted)?
Did the victim receive any threatening letters or other communications?
Did the victim receive any unsolicited gifts by mail for birthday or special holidays?
Was an unsolicited sample of a new product received in the mail?

[a]Aadapted from Crimes Involving Poison, Department of the Army Technical Bulletin PMG 21, 1967.

5.6.1. Product Tampering

There is always the possibility that the death was due to a tampered-with substance (food, drug, cosmetic, etc.). According to the Federal Anti-Tampering Act, it is a felony to tamper with foods, drugs, devices, cosmetics, and other consumer products. There are certain governmental agencies that now or in the past have been involved with the investigation of product tampering.

Prior to 1989, the FDA maintained the Elemental Analysis Research Center, in Cincinnati, Ohio, and in 1989, the FDA began the Forensic Chemistry Center, also located in Cincinnati.

What might have been the possible points of entry for contamination? Could it have been during the manufacturing process, at the hands of an employee, or a form of industrial sabotage?

Could it have been done during distribution of the product, when it was tampered with and returned to the shelf looking untouched (remember the "Poisoner Camouflage," where the offender has a specific victim in mind, and tries to make the crime look like a random death). Could the tampering have occurred after the point of purchase, which are usually false report cases wherein an individual is seeking some financial settlement from the manufacturer.

5.6.2. Analytical Toxicology

We now come to the part of the investigation in which a specialized form of chemical qualitative and quantitative analysis takes place. This is usually done in a forensic toxicology laboratory. The criminal investigator needs to remember that these analytical tests do not routinely test for all chemical substances. These laboratories normally have a set of specialized toxicology screens that they utilize. These general tests usually are: drug screens looking for commonly abused substances; *heavy metal screens* looking for substances such as arsenic, antimony, thallium, lead, etc.; and *volatile substance screens* looking for solvents such as chloroform or ether. There may also be *general analytical screens* that detect cyanide, volatiles, strychnine, heavy metals, and drugs.

Remember that when a result comes back negative, it means only that none of the substances tested for were present in detectable quantities, not that the specimen was free of all chemical substances. It would be nice if someday, like *Star Trek's* Dr.

McCoy, we could pass a "Tricorder" over the body in question and thereby scan for over a million different chemical entities. Such technology is too far in the future to be of help to us at present.

However, it is very possible for the criminal investigator and pathologist to be of great assistance to the team running the toxicological analyses, if they are aided by an indication of what substances are suspected. This help comes from the death scene investigation and any abnormalities found on autopsy. Remember, one can not find what one is not looking for.

It is also important to remember that the analytical work can only indicate the presence and possibly quantity of a poisonous material, but not the reason for the exposure. It is up to the death investigator to determine the reason for the exposure. One observation that might be helpful is that there can be differences in quantitative amount of the lethal material. In a homicide, usually just the right amount for a lethal dose is given, while in a suicide, usually a massive amount has been taken.

In order to carry out a proper toxicological analysis, the analyst must have the proper specimens. In gathering specimens for testing, one must be absolutely certain all specimen containers are clean and not contaminated, and that the proper chain of evidence has been maintained. For the specimens and amounts needed of each, please refer to **Table 5-2.**

5.6.3. Analysis of Cremated Remains

Although it would seem at first glance that the ashes of a deceased person could be analyzed for toxic substances, this does present some very definite analytical and legal problems.

First, many chemical substances will be burned off at the high temperatures required for cremation, which would yield a false negative result. Legally, one cannot prove that sample is pure, as it could be contaminated with other cremated remains; therefore the chain of evidence is broken. One would also not be able to prove that the poison was in systemic circulation and therefore caused the death. One would not be able to prove what organ the poison originated in, and therefore there would be no basis for comparison (e.g., mg of arsenic per g of liver). Although the analysis of cremated

Table 5-2
Desired Specimens for Toxicological Analyses

Urine (all available)
Gastric contents (all available)
Blood (heart = 25 mL, peripheral = 10 mL)
Brain (100 g)
Liver (100 g)
Kidney (50 g)
Bile (all available)
Vitreous humor (all available)
Hair/nails

remains were first used in the poisoning conviction of Graham Young in the UK in 1972, it would seem that this type of evidence has too many pitfalls to warrant its use.

The astute criminal investigator might begin to wonder if it is ever possible to detect murder by poison, and if there is anything that might serve to warn an investigator of the possibility. Some things that might come up in the investigation that should put up a red flag have been summarized in **Table 5-3**.

Certainly a person can die without warning, but when there is a sudden death in a normally healthy individual, a deeper look into the cause is called for, including an autopsy.

When an individual interferes with the victim receiving proper medical attention, one wonders if they do not want educated eyes and minds delving into the possible cause of the condition in question.

No signs of violence to the body is always an indication that the death could have been due to a poisoning misadventure.

When an illness reoccurred in cycles, that is, the victim became ill at home, went to a medical facility and seemed to recover, then went home and became ill again, and so on, this would indicate that there is something in the home environment that is proving unhealthy for the individual. Could it be the chronic administration of heavy metals (e.g., arsenic) with meals? There certainly have been recorded criminal cases where this has happened, and the poisoner is often not caught in the initial stages of the homicide attempt.

If there are common mysterious symptoms in a common group of people, it could indicate that there has been a mass tampering,

Table 5-3
When Should Suspicions Be Aroused?

Was it a sudden death in normally healthy individual?
Was there interference with receipt of proper medical attention?
Is there a lack of visible signs of violence to the body?
Was there a history of cyclical illness?
Are there mysterious symptoms in a common group of people?
Is there an individual anxious to dispose of food, drink, or medicine?
Were friends/relations prevented from being sent for during the illness?
Is there insistence on no autopsy?
Is there insistence on immediate cremation?
Are explanations being freely offered for cause of death?
Is someone attempting to guide your investigation?
Does any individual have a knowledge of poisons?

or that the supposed specific target was a little off the mark of the poisoner.

When there is an individual who is anxious to dispose of food, drink, or medicine of which the victim partook, it is clear that they are attempting to foil the investigation by the destruction of critical evidence.

If an individual prevented friends or relations from being sent for during the illness of the victim, one should question what they did not want others to witness.

If there is an insistence on no autopsy, the criminal investigator should clearly state that one will take place. Once again, the desire to have educated minds look at the problem comes to the forefront.

An insistence on a rapid cremation could be construed as an attempt to burn the primary evidence of the crime and foil the investigation. The criminal investigator should clearly state that an investigation must take place before cremation can proceed.

While grieving over the loss of a close family member or friend, most people will not freely begin to offer an explanation for the cause of death. Neither will they attempt to guide the investigation in any way. If they do, it could very well be an attempt to divert investigators' attention from their crime, and investigators must be aware of this.

If there is an individual who shows a familiarity with poisons, and literature about poisons, then not just a red flag should go up, but a whole sky full of mental fireworks.

5.7. HOW DID THE POISON GET IN THE PATIENT?

Once it has been determined by autopsy that poison was present in the victim, the question arises as to how the poisoning occurred.

It is possible that the cause was accidental. It could be present from a natural source, such as heavy metal contamination of ground water in the environment, or contamination of the body by leaching of heavy metals prior to exhumation. Another natural source is food or drink, such as the temporary elevation of arsenic levels often seen after a seafood meal. Elevated levels of poison, such as lead, can result from occupational exposures, such as shooting ranges, electroplating facilities, or smelters. There could also be a possible metabolic cause for the presence of the poison in the deceased, such as the elevated copper levels one sees with a condition known as "Wilson's Disease." It could be due to an error in the filling of a prescription with the wrong medication, or incorrect instructions, or it could have come from some contamination in the home environment, such as carbon monoxide.

The poison could have been self-administered, as in the case of the accidental misuse of a product, the unforeseen result of substance abuse, or the intent of the victim to commit suicide.

The poison might have been administered by another person, perhaps from product tampering or with homicidal intent.

In all, the poisoning crime scene is one surrounded by mystery and invisible clues. But when a criminal investigator begins to focus on the possibilities, the mysterious fog begins to clear a little, and the face of the poisoner becomes more visible.

Our ability to detect poisons has greatly improved over the last 100 years, but our ability to suspect poisoning in the first place has not improved, and may have actually gotten worse.

5.8. REFERENCES

Crimes Involving Poison. Department of the Army Technical Bulletin *TB PMG 21*, Department of the Army, Washington, D.C., 1967, pp. 11–13.

Sparrow G: *Women Who Murder*, Abelard-Schuman, New York, NY. 1970. p. 156.

5.9. SUGGESTED READINGS

Thorwald J: *The Century of the Detective*. Harcourt, Brace & World, New York, NY, 1964.

Thorwald J: *Crime and Science: The New Frontier in Criminology*. Harcourt, Brace & World, New York, NY, 1966.

Chapter 6

The Forensic Autopsy

During the autopsy, the forensic pathologist will be looking for certain clues that might indicate that a poison could have been involved in the death. These clues could include: irritated tissues (from caustic and corrosive compounds), characteristic odors, such as the almond-like odor of cyanide, or Mees lines (white bands on the nail that indicate chronic exposure to heavy metals like arsenic). The pathologist will also review the results of toxicological screens, to see if they are consistent with his pathological findings. Certain cautions in the interpretation of the analytical toxicology results should be observed.

The concentrations of substances revealed by an analytical test will vary depending on the site of origin of the specimen as well as the length of time that has passed since the initial exposure. The reliability of any postmortem specimen is directly related to the conditions associated with the collection of that specimen. It has become increasingly clear that blood concentrations of many drugs are definitely dependent on the site of collection, and that blood concentrations may be significantly higher, or sometimes lower, than at the time of death. For the pathologist to merely remove blood from the left side of the heart, or worse yet, obtain a sample from the chest or abdominal cavity of the victim, can yield results that may lead the investigators far astray from the actual meaningful and more accurate analytical results. Unfortunately, our ability to interpret the results of toxicological analyses has not kept pace with the great advancements that have been made in the detection limits of our analytical instrumentation.

It is unfortunate that the literature available on postmortem levels in fatal intoxications typically consists only of case reports. It would be of extreme value to forensic scientists if an international database existed listing chemical substances that have been detected in bodies in relation to the time interval since death. This database should list the name of the substance, the type of specimen, the time interval since death that the specimen was obtained as well as analyzed, the determined level, and the type of analytical technique utilized. In other words, how long after death was it possible to prove the presence of a substance in the body? This information has major implications when considering the possible value of exhuming the body of a victim thought to have been poisoned.

It is well known that chemical substances redistribute in the body, a phenomenon often referred to as *"anatomical site concentration"* or *"postmortem redistribution."* This phenomenon could also well be called *"necro-kinetics,"* or the movement of substances after death has occurred. Many studies have shown that certain drugs, such as propoxyphene and the tricyclic antidepressants, have an increase in heart blood concentrations postmortem. Some researchers have proposed that drug concentrations obtained from liver specimens are much better indicators of toxicity.

Factors that can alter the movement of substances, and therefore their final concentrations in an analytical specimen, include acid-base changes in the body after death and the *"volume of distribution"* (*Vd*) of the substance in question. Drugs with a low Vd will become less ionized as the pH in the body decreases (becomes more acidic), and therefore their solubility in the surrounding tissues will increase. Examples of drugs that will shift with this change in acidity include salicylates, theophylline, and phenobarbital.

The ideal toxicological sample would be a peripheral sample obtained from a blood vessel that had been ligated shortly after death. Unfortunately, this ideal is seldom obtained in the case of homicidal poisoning!

The following guidelines must be kept in mind when carrying out a toxicological analysis:

1. Postmortem concentrations are absolutely site-dependent.
2. Samples taken from the same site in the body will show different concentrations postmortem, depending on the time of obtaining the sample.

3. From a single postmortem measurement, no realistic calculation of the absorbed dose to create that level can really be made.
4. When obtaining samples for analysis a clean instrument must be used for each specimen to avoid possible cross-contamination of specimens and erroneous results.
5. Both the death scene investigator and the pathologist can provide crucial information to the toxicological analyst.
6. Absolute chain-of-custody, must be maintained on all specimens throughout the process from their procurement through their toxicological analyses.

REFERENCES

Druid H, Holmgren P: A compilation of fatal and control concentrations of drugs in postmortem femoral blood. *J Forensic Sci* 1997; 42(1):79–87.

Hilberg T, Rogde S, Morland J: Postmortem drug redistribution — human cases related to results in experimental animals. *J Forensic Sci* 1999; 44(1):3–9.

Imwinkelried EJ: Forensic science: toxicological procedures to identify poisons. *Crim Law Bull* 1994: 30:172–179.

Jones GR, Pounder DJ: Site dependence of drug concentrations in postmortem blood — a case study. *J Analy Toxicol* 1987; 11:187–191.

Langford AM, Pounder DJ: Possible markers for postmortem drug redistribution. *J Forensic Sci* 1997; 42(1):88–82.

Moriya F, Hashimoto Y: Redistribution of basic drugs into cardiac blood from surrounding tissues during early-states postmortem. *J Forensic Sci* 1999; 44(1):10–16.

Pounder DJ, Jones GR: Postmortem drug redistribution — a toxicological nightmare. *Forensic Sci International* 1990; 45:253–263.

Repetto MR, Repetto M: Habitual, toxic, and lethal concentrations of 103 drugs of abuse in humans. *Clin Tox* 1997; 35(1):1–9.

Repetto MR, Repetto M: Therapeutic, toxic, and lethal concentrations in human fluids of 90 drugs affecting the cardiovascular and hematipoietic systems. *Clin Tox* 1997; 35(4):345–351.

Repetto MR, Repetto M: Therapeutic, toxic and lethal concentrations of 73 drugs affecting respiratory system in human fluids. *Clin Tox* 1998; 36(4):287–293.

Repetto MR, Repetto M: Concentrations in human fluids: 101 drugs affecting the digestive system and metabolism. *Clin Tox* 1999; 37(1):1–8.

Watson WA: The toxicokinetics of poisoning and drug overdose. *Am Assoc Clin Chem* 1991 12(8):7–12.

Chapter 7

Proving Poisoning

> *"It is a capital mistake to theorize before one has data. Insensibly one begins to twist facts to suit theories, instead of theories to suit facts."*—Sherlock Holmes (by Sir Arthur Conan Doyle)

Let us begin our discussion of the proof that a murder by poison has been committed by discussing the proper utilization of the services of an analytical toxicology laboratory, because they will play a key role in the detection of the crime.

First of all, the "shot gun" approach to detection will most likely not be successful. One cannot hand them a specimen and say that poisoning is suspected, and ask them to prove that a poisonous compound is present in the specimen. The analysts need some guidelines as to what compounds are suspected. These guidelines will come from the criminal investigator's analysis of the death scene, as well as the pathological findings that will come from the autopsy. The key here is that once there has been a death, a qualified Medical Examiner should be called in to the case immediately.

The investigator should also be aware that the concentration of compounds may differ depending on the site of origin of a blood specimen, in that cardiac (heart) blood may differ from peripheral (away from the central portion) blood in the quantitative analyses.

7.1. KEY ELEMENTS TO BE PROVEN

1. Discovery consists of legally proving that a crime was committed, and demonstrating beyond reasonable doubt that death was caused by poison, administered with malicious or evil intent to the deceased. Never forget the importance of the chain of evidence on all investigational specimens.
2. Motive is critical because here the investigator must clearly establish the instigating force responsible for carrying out the action. Why would anyone want to carry out such an act on the victim? Here is where the close study of the victim ("victimology") becomes central to the case.
3. Intent constitutes the purpose or aim that an individual would have in commission of the act. Here the investigator will cover the desired outcome of the criminal act.
4. Access to the poison responsible for the death. In this area, the criminal investigator will present such evidence as proof of sale of the poison, with such things as receipts or the signature on a poison register at the point of sale. Are there any original packaging, wrappers, or containers associated to suspect? It may suffice to prove that a suspect has had access at a workplace, used toxins or poisons in his occupation, or had a hobby that involved the use of the poison in question.
5. Access to the victim. Proof that a suspect has knowledge of the victim's daily habits, could have had the opportunity to overcome any of the victim's normal defenses, and was able to administer the poison either directly or indirectly.
6. Death was caused by poison. There must be sufficient, sound evidence that would induce a reasonable person to come to this conclusion. Remember that in order to prove death by poison, the presence of the poison in the systemic circulation and/or body organs must be proven. The presence of the poison only in the gastrointestinal (GI) tract does not prove death by poisoning. The GI tract from mouth to anus is much like a garden hose: hollow and open at both ends, and therefore outside the topological framework of the body. Therefore, in order to meet its fatal potential, the poisonous compound must be absorbed through the walls of the gut and enter the body's systemic circulation.
7. The death was homicidal. This proof can not be done analytically or by autopsy, but depends on the work of the criminal investigator at

the crime scene, and examination of witnesses. This proof must categorically eliminate the possibility that the death resulted from an accident, intentional substance abuse, or an act of suicide.

In conclusion, it is imperative for the possibility of a conviction that these investigational proofs clearly lead to the conclusion that the death was caused by poison, that the accused administered the poison to the deceased, that no other person was possible or probable to have administered the substance, and that the accused was well aware of the poison's lethal effect on the victim.

7.2. STATISTICAL ANALYSES OF POISONINGS IN THE UNITED STATES

To the author's knowledge, no major epidemiological study has ever been done prior to the 1990s that reviews poisoning homicides in the United States. The first such study was carried out by Westveer, Trestrail, and Pinizotto, and was published in 1996. These investigators decided to look at the data contained in the Uniform Crime Reports (UCR), maintained by the Department of Justice, from 1980 to 1989. These reports, submitted annually from police agencies across the United States, provide some information on the victim and the offender in various crimes. This information includes: month; year; state; victim information (gender, age, and race); offender information (gender, age, and race); classification of poisonous agent as drug, nondrug, or fume; relationship between victim and offender; and a motive classification group. For this decade, a total of 202,785 homicides were reported, and in this compilation of all homicides, there were 292 poisoning cases of a single offender on a single victim. This total represents 14 poisoning cases per 10,000 homicides. The following information was determined from a statistical analysis of the UCR data.

Gender relationships:

- The victims equally divided between male and female.
- If the victim was a female, the offender was usually a male.
- If the victim was a male, the offender could have been equally male or female.
- Offenders were male twice as often as female.

Racial relationships:

- The victim and offender were usually of the same race.
- The victims were mostly white.
- If the victim was white, the offender was usually male.
- If the victim was black, the offender was equally male or female.
- Black victims were males twice as often as females.
- White victims were equally male or female.
- For black or white offenders, there were twice as many males as females.

Age characteristics:

- Victims were highest in the 25–29 years of age range.
- Offenders were highest in the 20–34 years of age range.

Geographical relationships:

- Poisonings average 1.47 per million people per year.
- Poisoning were highest in the Western region; the state of California has the highest number.

Other relationships:

- Probably one of the most startling revelations from this study was that the unknown offender rate for poisoning cases was 20–30 times higher than nonpoisoning homicides. This would seem to indicate that a poisoning was determined to be the cause of death, yet no offender was ever found. This is another indication for law enforcement, and other forensic scientists, to sharpen their investigative skills in the area of murder by poison.
- More victims were of a relationship outside the offender's family. This is an unusual result, as it would seem that most homicidal poisonings are a crime of the domestic environment.
- Nondrug poisons were used by 50% more males than females, and drug poisons were used by three times as many males as females.
- Poisoning rate by year or month was relatively constant. There was no month or year that showed a significant increase or decrease in the number of poisoning cases reported.

The next parts of this study will look at the data that represents poisoning cases in which a single offender poisoned multiple victims—the serial poisoner—and the relatively rare cases that represent multiple offenders on a single victim.

7.3. REFERENCES

Doyle AC: "A Scandal in Bohemia," In: *The Complete Sherlock Holmes*, Doubleday & Co., Inc., Garden City, NY, 1930, p. 163.

Westveer AE, Trestrail JH, Pinizzoto J: Homicidal poisonings in the United States—An analysis of the Uniform Crime Reports from 1980 through 1989. *Amer J. Foren Med Path*, 1996;17(4):282–288.

7.4. SUGGESTED READING

Browne GL, Stewart CG: *Reports of Trials for Murder by Poisoning*. Stevens and Sons, London, 1883.

Chapter 8

POISONERS IN COURT

> *"Revolted by the odious crime of homicide, the chemist's aim is to perfect the means of establishing proof of poisoning so that the heinous crime will be brought to light and proved to the magistrate who must punish the criminal."* —Traite de Poison, M. J. B. Orfila (1814)

The majority of the death scene investigation has been completed. Evidence has been gathered that points to a defendant as the probable perpetrator of a murder by means of poison. It is now time to take the evidence that proves method, motive, and opportunity to the jury. Let's take a look at some of the differences that might be encountered in the poisoning trial vs trials for murder by means of more traditional weapons.

8.1. BATTERY BY POISON

One may commit a battery by causing injury through poisoning. Battery, of course, occurs when a person is injured in a dangerous situation intentionally created by the defendant.

A defendant is held to be culpable in a battery charge if he/she acts with either an intent to injure or with criminal negligence. "Aggravated battery" is punishable as a felony, and results from actions taken with the intent to kill. In this case, usually the defendant must have intended to cause the specific result; otherwise the crime is considered a "regular battery" charge.

8.2. STANDARD DEFENSE ARGUMENTS

When the poisoner goes on trial, obtaining a conviction will be far from simple. It is at this point that the results of the investigator's careful and detailed work will become critical. In this section, we will attempt to discuss some prosecution strategies and defense tactics that might come into play.

Unlike trials where murder has been carried out by means of a visibly detectable weapon (e.g., gun, knife, rope), in the trial for murder by poison, one must not forget that the vast majority of the trial evidence will be indirect evidence, or circumstantial evidence. In the poisoning crime, there will be few, if any, witnesses.

The defendant will attempt to explain the facts being presented by the prosecutor. The poisoner's best defense is the simplest answer that explains the facts. Among some of the possible counterarguments that will be attempted by the defense team are the following:

8.2.1. Poisoning Not the Cause of Death

The defense will attempt to prove that the poison did not cause the death, but that the victim died from another cause. For example, the defense might argue that the cause of death was due to a subdural hematoma from a fall, and not from the effects of a poison. At this point, the detailed work combination of forensic pathologist and analytical toxicologist will come into play.

8.2.2. Poisoning Not *Homicidal*

The defendant will attempt to downplay his involvement in the death, by trying to convince the court that the victim caused his/her death by self-administering the poison, either with suicidal intent or as the fatal result of substance abuse.

8.2.3. No Homicidal Intent

It could be suggested that the substance was administered by the accused, but not with the intent to murder. One is reminded of the Arthur Ford case in the UK, discussed in Chapter 1, in which the offender administered candy containing Cantharides in order to arouse sexually two secretaries in his office. He was convicted of manslaughter, because the court agreed that his intent was not to kill. Another case would be the unfortunate death of comedian John Belushi from an overdose of drugs administered by another person.

8.2.4. Substance **Not** *a Poison*

Legal experts will argue over the acceptable definition of a "poison." Is it a drug, and not a poison? Remember Paracelsus' definition of a poison: that it is solely related to dose. The major factors that determine the potential lethality of any substance are concentration and duration of exposure. This was clearly stated in 1915 by the German chemist Fritz Haber, who developed what was known as the "ct product." His formula was $c \times t = a$ constant. What this means is that the product of the concentration of a poison and the survival time of the victim is a constant. For example, breathing a certain concentration of carbon monoxide for a specified amount of time will produce the same effects as breathing one-half the concentration for twice the time—the toxicological result should be a constant outcome.

8.2.5. Accused Had a Reason to Have the Poison in His/Her Possession

As to why the accused had the poisonous substance in his/her possession, it will be argued that it was acceptably associated with his job (e.g., chemist) or hobby (e.g., photography), or that the substance was being used as a domestic pesticide to rid the area of unwanted pests (rodents, insects, weeds, fungi, etc.).

8.3. PROBLEMS PROVING INTENTIONAL POISONING

The attorney for the prosecution is bound to find him or herself beset with some rather unique problems in a poisoning trial. One of the major problems is that the majority of the evidence will be circumstantial (indirect). In the typical murder by poison, there will be no witnesses to the act. Another problem is that there may not be an accepted legal definition of a poison. There is also bound to be a great

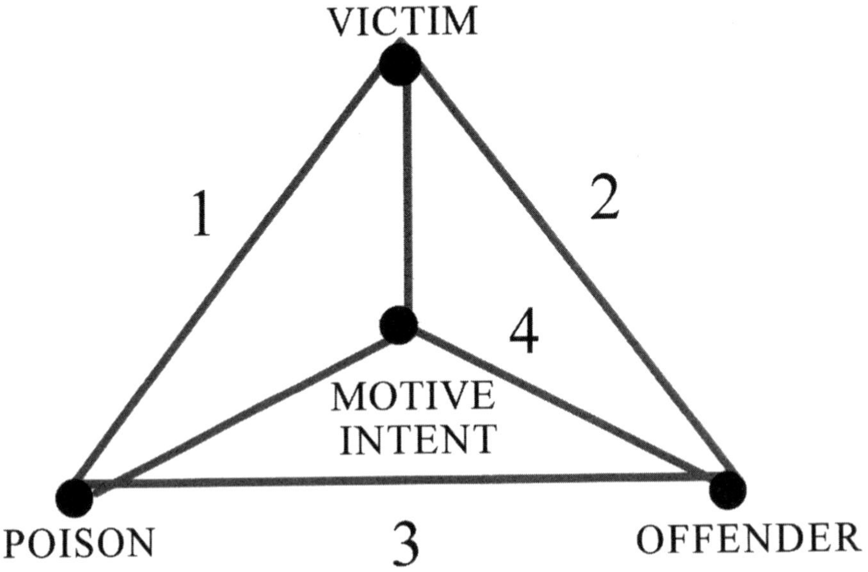

deal of dispute over the scientific evidence, and much of the evidence is likely to be rebutted by other technical experts.

The goal in obtaining a conviction is to prove that the death was caused by a poison, hopefully with a combination of pathological and analytical evidence. It must be proven that the accused administered the poison because he/she had the access, and opportunity, and that it is not possible or probable that any other person could have administered the substance. It is also imperative to prove that the accused was aware of the poison's lethality.

Is would be wise for the prosecution to prepare their case while keeping in mind what the author has named the "Conviction Pyramid" (*see* **Fig. 8-1**). This concept represents the four major points that must proven to be connected in the case: Victim, Poison, Poisoner, and Motive. Unless each of these points is linked together, there may be trouble in obtaining a conviction.

The case usually begins with the discovery of the two points representing leg 1, *Victim-Poison,* but the proofs must also encompass the more difficult legs of the Conviction Pyramid numbered 2, 3, and 4: *Offender-Victim, Offender-Poison,* and *Motive/Intent-Offender*. Unless each of these points is unquestionably linked, there may be great difficulty in obtaining a conviction.

Table 8-1
The Poisoner Equation

1. Poison **X** is found in **B.**
2. **A** had motive for elimination of **B**.
3. **A** had access to **X** by purchase or theft.
4. **A** had knowledge of poison **X**.
5. Container of **X** found in the possession of **A**.
6. **A** had access to **B**.
7. Therefore, **A** poisoned **B**.

Adapted from Glaister, 1954

Laying out the poisoning case comes down to trying to solve the following algebraic equation, represented in **Table 8-1,** where **A** = plaintiff, **B** = victim, **X** = the poison.

Always remember the logic argument, which is known as "Occam's Razor," that the simplest solution to a problem is probably the correct one.

As one can see, the poisoning trial is beset with unique conviction pitfalls, but with proper investigational research, proper chain of evidence, and detailed planning, the chances of a conviction are greatly increased.

8.4. REFERENCES

Glaister J: *The Power of Poison*. William Morrow and Company, New York, NY, 1954.

Orfila MJB: *Traite de Poisons,* Chez Crochard, Paris, 1814

8.5. SUGGESTED READING

Boos WF: *The Poison Trail*. Hale, Cushman & Flint, Boston, 1939.

Notable British Trial Series (W. Hodge & Co., UK)

Trial of H.R. Armstrong, ed. by Filson Young.
Trial of Adelaide Bartlett, ed. by Sir John Hall.
Trial of George Chapman, ed. by H.L. Adam, 1930.
Trial of Neill Cream, ed. by W. Teignmouth Shore, 1923.
Trial of H. H. Crippen, ed. by Filson Young, 1920.
Trial of Harold Greenwood, ed. by Winifred Duke, 1930.
Trial of Dr. Lamson, ed. by H. L. Adam, 1913.

Trial of Mrs. Maybrick, ed by H. B. Irving, 1912.
Trial of William Palmer, ed. by G. H. Knott, 1912.
Trial of Dr. Pritchard, ed. by William Roughead, 1906.
Trial of The Seddons, ed. by Filson Young, 1914.
Trial of Madelaine Smith, ed. by A. Duncan Smith, 1905.
Trial of Madelaine Smith, ed. by F. Tennyson Jesse, 1927.

Chapter 9

Poisoning in Fiction

MARTHA: "Well, dear, for a gallon of elderberry wine, I take one teaspoonful of arsenic, and add a half a teaspoonful of strychnine, and then just a pinch of cyanide."—Arsenic and Old Lace, Joseph Kesselring

It is often said that life can imitate art, and so it would behoove us to look at the use of poisons in fictional works, both written and visual. The scenario of an individual reading a novel or watching a film, and obtaining ideas that could lead to committing an actual murder, is not beyond the realm of possibility.

In an attempt to gather some information on how poisons have been used in fiction, the author analyzed 187 fictional works to determine the types of poisons that had been used. They varied a little from those that have been actually used in cases of murder, but the primary ones did appear. In fiction, cyanide was used more often than was arsenic. The poisons used in fictional writings have been summarized in **Table 9-1.**

It is also important to look at the visual media as well, as there are some movies that can create ideas in the fertile mind of an individual. Some of the films that have used poisons in their plots are summarized in **Table 9-2**.

Table 9-1
Poisons Used in Literature (A Review of 187 Works)

Poison	# Cases	%
Acid	1	0.5%
Aconite	2	1.1%
Air (by injection)	1	0.5%
Akee	1	0.5%
Antimony	1	0.5%
Arrow poison	1	0.5%
Arsenic	13	7.0%
Atropine	5	2.7%
Barbitone	3	1.3%
Bowl cleaner	1	0.5%
Carbon monoxide	3	1.6%
Chloral	1	0.5%
Chloral hydrate	2	1.1%
Coal gas	2	1.1%
Cocaine	2	1.1%
Coniine	1	0.5%
Curare	4	2.1%
Cyanea capillata	1	0.5%
Cyanide	25	13.4%
"Devil's Foot Root"	1	0.5%
Digitalin	3	1.6%
Digitalis	3	1.6%
Digitoxin	1	0.5%
Drugs	1	0.5%
Fear: of poison death	2	1.1%
Food poisoning	1	0.5%
Formic acid	1	0.5%
Fungus	1	0.5%
Gelsemium	1	0.5%
Hemlock	1	0.5%
Henbane	1	0.5%
Hexabarbital	1	0.5%
Hyoscine	3	1.6%
Indian Hemp + *Datura*	1	0.5%
Jimson Weed	2	1.1%
L-thyroxine	1	0.5%
Microorganisms: Cholera	1	0.5%
Morphine	6	3.2%
Multiple poisons	1	0.5%

(table 9-1 continued)

Poison	# Cases	%
Muscarine	1	0.5
Mushrooms	15	8.0
Narcotic	1	0.5
Nicotine	6	3.2
Nitrobenzene	2	1.1
Oleander	2	1.1
Paint thinner	1	0.5
Phenylbutazone allergy	1	0.5
Phosphorus	1	0.5
Photographic developer	1	0.5
Physostigmine	2	1.1
Poison gas	1	0.5
Poisoned darts	1	0.5
Procaine	1	0.5
Purvisine (an alkaloid)	1	0.5
Ricin	2	1.1
Serenite (an invented poison)	1	0.5
Solanine	1	0.5
Strptomycin allergy	1	0.5
Strophanthin	5	2.7
Strychnine	6	3.2
Taxine	1	0.5
Tetra-ethyl-pyrophosphate	1	0.5
Tetrodotoxin	1	0.5
Thallium	2	1.1
Toxin	1	0.5
Trinitrin	1	0.5
Tuberculin	1	0.5
Unidentified native poison	2	1.1
Unknown poison	13	7.0
Venom: bee	2	1.1
Venom: snake	4	2.1
Virus	1	0.5
Warfarin	1	0.5
Total	187	100.0

As part of the investigation of a criminal poisoning, it would be wise for the investigator to also look into fictional literature and visual media to which the suspect had access.

Table 9-2
Poisons Used in Motion Pictures (A Review of 15 Works)

Film title	Date	Poison used
Attack of the Mushroom People	1964	Mushrooms
Beguiled, The	1971	Mushrooms
Black Widow	1987	Penicillin allergy+unknowns
Court Jester, The	1956	Unknown
Dead Pool, The	1988	Street drug
D.O.A.	1949	Iridium
D.O.A.	1988	Radium chloride
Fer-de-Lance	1974	Venom: snake
Flesh and Fantasy	1943	Aconite
Goliath Awaits	1981	Algae extract ("Palmer's Disease")
Pope of Greenwich Village, The	1984	Lye (Sodium hydroxide)
Serpent and the Rainbow, The	1988	Tetrodotoxin
Throw Mama from the Train	1987	Lye (Sodium hydroxide)
Venom	1982	Venom: snake
Young Sherlock Holmes	1985	Dart poison

REFERENCES

Bardell EB: Dame Agatha's dispensary. *Pharmacy In History*, 1984;26(1):13–19.

Bond RT: Handbook for Poisoners: *Handbook for Poisoners: A Collection of Great Poison Stories.* Rinehart & Co., New York, NY, 1951.

Corvasce MV, Paglino JR: Modus Operandi: *A Writer's Guide to How Criminals Work.* The Howdunit Series, Writer's Digest Books, Cincinnati, OH, 1995.

Done AK: History of poisons in opera. *Mithridata* (newsletter of the Toxicological History Society), 1992;2(2):3–13.

Foster N: Strong poison: Chemistry in the works of Dorothy L. Sayers, in: *Chemistry and Crime:* (Gerber SM ed.), American Chemical Society, Washington, DC, 1983;17–29.

Gerald MC: *The Poisonous Pen of Agatha Christie.* University of Texas Press, Austin, TX, 1993.

Gwilt JR: Brother Cadfael's herbiary. *Pharmaceutical Journal,* December 19/26, 1992;807–809.

Gwilt PR: Dame Agatha's poisonous pharmacopoeia. *Pharmaceutical Journal,* 1978; 28,30:572–573.

Gwilt PR, et al. The use of poison in detective fiction. *Clue: A Journal of Detection,* 1981;1:8–17.

Kasselring J: *Arsenic and Old Lace,* New York Pocket Books, New York, NY, 1944.

Reinert RE: There ARE toadstools in murder mysteries (part I). *Mushroom Journal of Wild Mushrooming,* 1991–92;5–10.

Reinert RE: There ARE toadstools in murder mysteries (Part II). *Mushroom Journal of Wild Mushrooming,* 1994;12(2):9–12.

Reinert RE: More mushrooms in mystery stories. *Mushroom Journal of Wild Mushrooming*, 1996–97;15(1):5–7.
Stevens SD, Klarner A: *Deadly Doses: A Writer's Guide to Poisons.* The Howdunit Series, Writer's Digest Books, Cincinnati, OH, 1990.
Tabor E: Plant poisons in Shakespeare. *Economic Botany*, 1970;24:81–94.
Thompson CJS: Poisons in fiction, in: *Poison Mysteries in History, Romance, and Crime.* J.B. Lippincott, Philadelphia, 1924;254–261.

SUGGESTED READING

Winn D: *Murder Ink: The Mystery Reader's Companion.* Workman Publishing, New York, NY, 1977.
Winn D: *Murderess Ink: The Better Half of the Mystery.* Workman Publishing, New York, NY, 1979.

Chapter 10

Conclusion

> *"If all those buried in our cemeteries who were poisoned could raise their hand, we would probably be shocked by the numbers!"*
> — (John Trestrial)

As Sir Arthur Conon Doyle's Sherlock Holmes in "The Adventure of Abbey Grange" stated to his partner Dr. Watson, "The game is afoot..." and so it is with investigators and the criminal poisoner. As homicide investigators, and now hopefully dedicated "Toxic Avengers," we must remember that unless we remain ever vigilant, we will lose the catch-the-poisoner game. Unless the possibility of poisoning is considered initially, the critical evidence of the crime will most likely be buried with the victim, and the poisoner will escape prosecution feeling both intellectually superior and smug.

The *Prime Directive* for any criminal investigation is that *every death must be considered a homicide until the facts prove otherwise!* To this we must now add a new *Sub-Directive* for the criminal investigation of homicidal poisonings: *Every death with no visible signs of trauma must be considered a poisoning until the facts prove otherwise!*

The investigative key is to put all the clues together, and where they overlap, one should be able to match the most prob-

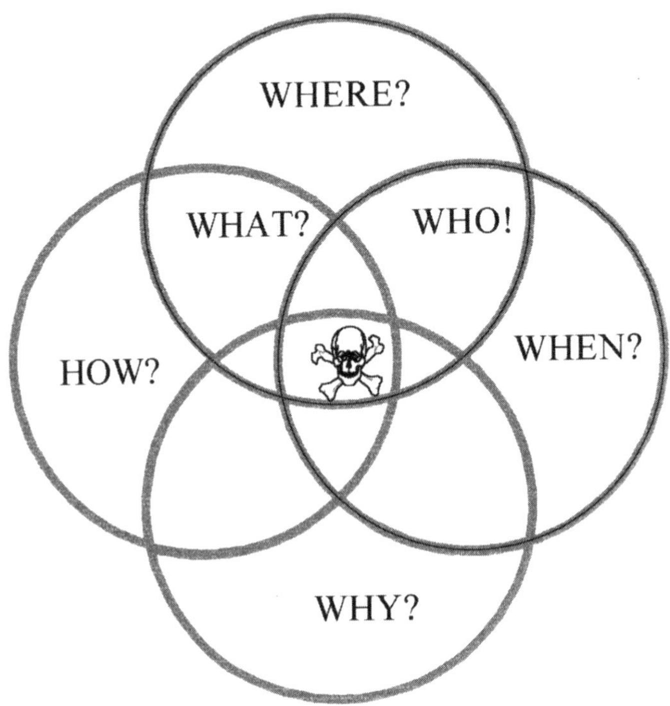

able offender. Let's review the basic categories of clues as they relate to poisoning homicides (*see* **Fig. 10-1**).

WHO was the victim, a specific or random target? Could a camouflaged poisoner be hiding behind a tampering? Why would anyone want to kill this individual, as determined by "victimology?"

WHAT was the poison weapon? Whether it is solid, liquid, or gas, poisons are just atoms and molecules that carry out their biochemical destruction in the manner of a "chemical monkey wrench." It is imperative that the poison be proven to have been in the victim's systemic circulation.

WHERE did the crime take place? A poisoning may have multiple crime scenes (procurement, preparation, administration, disposal, and ultimately the death scene).

WHEN was the poison administered to the victim? The time from administration till death is dependent on the concentration and toxicity of the substance. With an acute dose, one sees sudden onset. Analysis should be carried out on blood, urine, and

gastric contents (BUG). Look for poisons that have a rapid action (e.g., cyanide, strychnine, and so on). With a chronic dose situation, look for prolonged symptoms. Analysis should be carried out on the victim's hair to check for heavy metals (e.g., arsenic, antimony, lead, thallium, and so on).

WHY did the offender feel that the victim must be eliminated? What goal did the victim prevent the offender from achieving?

HOW was the poison administered? Look at the items used routinely and solely by the victim. The bottom line is that if investigators do not consider poisoning they will never detect it. The entire purpose of this important reference work can be summarized into a single graphic representation as seen above (*see* **Fig. 10-2**).

And now a concluding poetic challenge, from the poisoner to the newly educated *"Toxic Avengers."*

"The Poisoner"
by
John H. Trestrail III, RPh, FAACT, DABAT

The Borgias, DeMedicis and all those past—
you may have thought you had seen the last.
But we poisoners are still around today.
And if you miss my crime, I'll get away.
The body lies there neat and clean,
as the cause of death is seldom seen.
And the coroner may take time to pause—
is this death due to a natural cause?"
An autopsy or tox screen may reveal death's why,
but I hope the case will just slip by.
My crime is quiet and well thought through.
For you're used to violence—can I fool you?
The event's rarity is on my side,
For I count on you burying my homicide.
And though I roam free 'round the nation,
I live in fear of an exhumation.
The clues I leave may be hard to find,
you see, to me, I have a superior mind.
My weapons are there before your eyes,
but they are so very small—of molecular size.
I don't think you'll have a notion,
for mine is murder in slow motion.
It gives me time to just slip by,
and create my perfect alibi.
Where to look for me isn't clear.
I may be far, or I may be near.
I could be a stranger, though it is quite rare,
for I'm probably related to the victim there.
I chose the place, the means, and time,
for poisoning is usually a household crime.
The knowledge gained by my living close,
made it so very easy to deliver the dose.
Seeing it as poisoning would be profound,
but I think you'll miss it as you look around.
I'm a different kind of killer as you can see.
I am a POISONER—can you catch me?

"If all those buried in our cemeteries who were poisoned could raise their hand, we would probably be shocked by the numbers!"

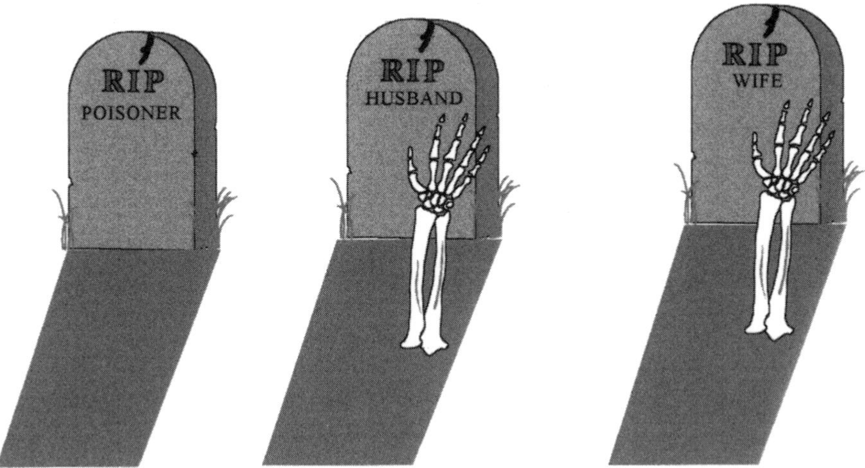

Appendix: Common Homicidal Poisons

ARSENIC

Form: Metallic arsenic (As) is a steel-gray, brittle metal. Arsenic trichloride ($AsCl_3$) is an oily liquid. Arsenic trioxide (As_2O_3) is a crystalline solid. It can also exist as arsine gas (AsH_3). Lewisite, a war gas, is a derivative of arsine.

Color: Metal (steel-gray), salts (white powder).

Odor: Odorless, but arsenic can produce a garlicky odor to the breath.

Solubility: Arsenical salts are water-soluble.

Taste: Almost tasteless.

Source: Pesticides, rodent poison, ant poison, homeopathic medications, weed killers, marine (copper arsenate) and other paints, ceramics, livestock feed.

Lethal Dose: Acute, 200 mg (As_2O_3); chronic, unknown.

How it Kills: Arsenic is a general protoplasmic poison; it combines with sulfhydral (-*SH*) groups on enzymes to inhibit their normal function. This results in disruption of normal metabolic pathways related to energy transfer.

Poison Notes: The trivalent arsenic (As^{+3}) is *more* toxic than the pentavalent (As^{+5}) form. Arsenic is one of the oldest poisons used by humans.

VICTIM OF ARSENIC

Administered: Often administered to victim in food or drink.

Symptom Onset Time Interval: Hours to days.

Symptoms–Acute: GI (30 minutes to 2 hours post-exposure): vomiting, bloody diarrhea, severe abdominal pain, burning esophageal pain, metallic taste in the mouth. Later symptoms include: jaundice, kidney failure, and peripheral neuropathies (destruction of the nervous system). Death from circulatory failure within 24 hours to 4 days.

Symptoms–Chronic: GI (diarrhea, abdominal pain), skin (hyperpigmentation of palms and soles), nervous system (symmetrical sensory neuropathy with numbness and loss of vibratory or positional sense, burning pain on the soles of the feet), localized edema (face, ankles), sore throat, stomatitis, pruritis, cough, tearing, salivation, garlic odor on breath, Aldrich-Mees lines (horizontal white lines that normally take 5 to 6 weeks to appear after the exposed nail bed area grows), hair loss.

Disease Confusion: Gastroenteritis, neurological disease.

Victim Notes: In homicides the amount of arsenic could be administered in a single large acute dose, or in frequent, small chronic doses to make the symptoms appear like a progressing natural illness. In suicides, the amount of arsenic taken is usually large.

DETECTION OF ARSENIC

Specimens: Food, beverages, medications, blood, urine, gastric contents, hair, nails, autopsy organ specimens.

Method: Colorimetric, atomic absorption (AA).

Toxic Levels:

Blood	Urine	Gastric	Other
0.6–9.3 mg/L	3,300 mcg/L	Unknown	3 ppm (hair/nails)
			>1 mcg/gm dry weight

Analysis Notes: Arsenic can be detected in hair and bones many years after poisoning. Several hairs pulled out by the root should be sent for analysis, with a clear indication of which end of the hair is the root. Segmented hair analysis using neutron activation gives an indication of arsenic exposure over the last several months.

SELECTED ARSENIC HOMICIDE CASES

Mary Blandy (1752)
Madeline Smith (1857)
Florence Maybrick (1889)
Johann Hoch (1905)
Henry Seddon (1911)
Mabel Greenwood (1919)
Herbert Armstrong (1921)
Michael Swango (1985)
Marie Hilley (1986)
Blanche Moore (1988)

BOTULINUS TOXIN

Form: Usually in the liquid form from culture medium.

Color: Colorless.

Odor: Odorless.

Solubility: Water-soluble.

Taste: Tasteless.

Source: Produced by the bacteria *Clostridium botulinum.*

Lethal Dose: Estimated to be as little as 0.1 mL of contaminated food. This substance is the most toxic known! The toxin is 7,000,000 times more lethal than cobra venom. Acute, 50 ng; chronic, not applicable.

How it Kills: Botulinus toxin irreversibly binds to cholinergic nerve terminals and prevents the release of acetylcholine (ACh) from the axon. Severe muscle weakness results, and subsequently death from respiratory failure.

Poison Notes: The toxin can grow in home-canned food at a pH of >4.5.

VICTIM OF BOTULINUS TOXIN

Administered: Could be administered in cool food or drink. Heating to a boiling temperature destroys the toxin within a few minutes.

Symptom Onset Time Interval: May be slow to onset (2 hours to 14 days). Death may occur as early as 10 hours after the symptoms first appear.

Symptoms–Acute: Dry sore throat, dry mouth, dizziness, vomiting, stomach upset, difficulty in swallowing, difficulty in speaking, double vision, drooping eye lids, cranial nerve weakness, progressive symmetric descending paralysis, and respiratory arrest.

Symptoms–Chronic: Not applicable.

Disease Confusion: Viral illness, Guillain-Barre syndrome, stroke, tick paralysis, heavy metal poisoning, adverse drug reactions, and many other conditions.

Victim Notes: None.

DETECTION OF BOTULINUS TOXIN

Specimens: Diagnosis is confirmed by determination of the toxin in serum, stool, or wound, and food, beverages, medications, blood, urine, and gastric contents. The test may be negative if the samples were collected late or the quantity of the toxin is small!

Method: Analysis is usually carried out by local health departments, or the CDC in Atlanta, GA.

Toxic Levels:

Blood	Urine	Gastric	Other
Not applicable	Not applicable	Not applicable	Not applicable

SELECTED BOTULINUS TOXIN HOMICIDE CASES

No cases on record.

CYANIDE

Form: In liquid form, hydrogen cyanide (HCN) is also known as "prussic acid." Pure hydrogen cyanide is a gas usually made by mixing an acid with cyanide salts. It is more commonly found in the form of sodium, potassium, or calcium salts, which are crystalline materials. Industrial cyanide can take the form of large nuggets called "cyanide eggs."

Color: Sodium and potassium salts of HCN are white.

Odor: Supposed to elicit the odor of almonds to some persons. (Note: 40–60% of the population cannot detect the odor because of a genetic difference—a form of "odor blindness.")

Solubility: Salts of cyanide are easily dissolved in aqueous liquids. Acidic liquids would cause the release of some HCN gas.

Taste: Salts of cyanide have a bitter (alkaline) taste, and can have a mild corrosive action on tissues.

Source: Fumigants, insecticides, rodenticides, metal polishes (especially silver polish), electroplating solutions, metallurgy for the extraction of gold and silver from ore, photographic processing, jewelers, and chemical laboratories. Contained as cyanogenic glycosides inside the pits and seeds of certain plants of genus *Prunus* (e.g., cherry, peach, bitter almonds, cassava, Laetrile, and so on). Cyanide can also be produced by the action of flame on the synthetic plastic materials polyurethane and polyacrylonitrile. It is also found as part of the intravenous antihypertensive drug molecule sodium nitroprusside (Nipride®). Cyanide is used in the most commonly employed method of synthesizing phencylidine (PCP).

Lethal Dose: Acute, 270 ppm (air), 50 mg (HCN), 200–300 mg (NaCN or KCN); chronic, unknown in all forms.

How it Kills: Cyanide shuts down respiration at the cellular level by inactivating essential enzymes, resulting in metabolic asphyxiation. Critical effects are on those organs most sensitive to oxygen deprivation, the brain and heart.

Poison Notes: Extreme care must be taken in providing mouth-to-mouth respiration support to victim, to avoid contamination of the individual providing aid.

VICTIM OF CYANIDE

Administered: Often administered to victim in food or drink.

Symptom Onset Time Interval: Immediate (as little as 30 seconds). Few poisons are as rapidly lethal.

Symptoms–Acute: Headache, nausea, vomiting, difficult breathing, and confusion. These initial symptoms are rapidly followed by seizures, coma, gasping respirations, and cardiovascular collapse.

Symptoms–Chronic: Not applicable.

Disease Confusion: Heart attack, acute asthmatic attack.

Victim Notes: An abrupt onset of profound symptoms after exposure is classic for cyanide exposure.

DETECTION OF CYANIDE

Specimens: Food, beverages, medications, blood, urine, gastric contents, and autopsy organ specimens.

Method: Colorimetric techniques.

Toxic Levels:

Blood	Urine	Gastric	Other
12.4 mg/L	0.1 mg/L	Unknown	Unknown

Analysis Notes: Toxic levels of cyanide in tissues may diminish significantly after death by mechanisms that include evaporation, thiocyanate formation, and reaction with tissue components. The formation of cyanide in postmortem tissues with accumulation to toxicologically significant levels apparently from the conversion of thiocyanate to cyanide has been demonstrated, but can be prevented by the addition of sodium fluoride (NaF). Blood specimens should be kept at temperatures from 20° to 4°F to reduce losses.

SELECTED CYANIDE HOMICIDE CASES

Theodosius Boughton (1781)
Dr. Collidge (1847)
Mrs. MacFarland (1911)
Twigg/Elosser (1911)
Jessie Costello (1933)
Ronald O'Bryan (1974)
People's Temple/Rev. Jim Jones (1978)
Tylenol tampering (Chicago) (1982)
Donald Harvey (1987)
Stella Nickel (1988)

SODIUM FLUOROACETATE

Form: Looks like flour or baking soda. Sodium fluoroacetate (a.k.a. sodium monofluoroacetate [SMFA], Furatol, Ratbane *1080*, or "Compound *1080*".) Sodium fluoroacetamide (a.k.a. Fluorakil, Fussol, Megarox) ancock, or "Compound *1081*"). It is also the toxic constituent of the South Africa plant Giftblaar (*Dichapetalum cymosum*).

Color: White, crystalline compound.

Odor: Odorless.

Solubility: *1080* is very water soluble, but has a low solubility in ethanol.

Taste: *1080* is mostly tasteless, but very dilute solutions may have a vinegar-like taste due to the acetate component.

Source: Pesticides, rodent poison, insect poison, and predator (coyote) poison. NOTE: it is sold only to licensed pest-control operators and others qualified by training and experience in rodent-control procedures. It is usually mixed with black dye and added to grain baits.

Lethal Dose: Acute, 2–10 mg/kg, 700 mg/150 lb victim; chronic, not applicable.

How it Kills: The salt's metabolite, fluorocitrate, blocks normal enzyme mechanisms in the body, acting mainly on the heart and central nervous system.

Poison Notes: As little as 1 mg of *1080* is sufficient to cause serious poisoning. This is one of the most toxic substances known, and there is no specific antidote.

VICTIM OF SODIUM FLUOROACETATE

Administered: *1080* can be administered to the victim in food or drink. It can also be absorbed through broken skin.

Symptom Onset Time Interval: Symptoms are delayed while the body converts the compound to the more toxic metabolite. Compound *1080*: from 30 minutes to several hours. Compound *1081*: slower onset of symptoms.

Symptoms–Acute: Nausea, vomiting, diarrhea, agitation, confusion, seizures, lethargy, coma, respiratory arrest, and cardiac arrhythmias.

Symptoms–Chronic: Not applicable.

Disease Confusion: Gastroenteritis, viral infection, heart attack.

DETECTION OF SODIUM FLUOROACETATE

Specimens: Blood, urine, and gastric contents.

Method: Specific gas chromatographic procedures for the identification of fluoroacetate in biological specimens have relied on flame-ionization, electron capture, or mass spectrometric detection of a derivative. There has been a report for a method for high-pressure liquid chromatography (HPLC) on gastric contents.

Toxic Levels:

Blood	Urine	Gastric	Other
Unknown	65 mg/L	12 mg/L	Liver: 58 mg/kg

SELECTED SODIUM FLUOROACETATE HOMICIDE CASES

No cases of record.

STRYCHNINE

Form: Strychnine is an alkaloidal plant compound obtained from the tree *Strychnos nux-vomica*. The seeds are discs (1-inch in diameter, 0.25-inch thick at the rim), with a central depression, gray-green color, and a satin-like appearance. Pure strychnine alkaloid is a white powder.

Color: White, crystalline powder.

Odor: None that is characteristic.

Solubility: Soluble in aqueous solutions.

Taste: Strychnine is extremely bitter, with a taste that is detectable at a dilution of 1:100,000. Strychnine could be administered in alcohol if the victim is accustomed to bitter drinks (e.g., tonic water). Strychnine can also be introduced into foods that normally have a sour or bitter taste.

Source: Rodenticides (concentrations over 0.5% are currently distributed only to licensed exterminators). Sometimes found as an adulterant in illicit drugs. At one time, strychnine was sold over the counter as an ingredient in a variety of stimulant tonics and laxatives.

Lethal Dose: Acute, 5–8 mg/kg, 30–100 mg (oral); chronic, unknown.

How it Kills: Respiratory arrest.

VICTIM OF STRYCHNINE

Administered: Food, beverages, medications.

Symptom Onset Time Interval: 15–30 minutes (oral route), 5 minutes (IV or nasal route).

Symptoms–Acute: Muscle stiffness and painful cramps, which precede generalized muscle contractions. The victim's body may take the form of an arch (with only head and heels touching the floor)—this is called an "opisthotonic" convulsion. The face may be drawn into a forced smile or sardonic grin called *risus sardonicus*. The muscle contractions (spasms) are intermittent and can be easily triggered by emotional or physical stimuli (sound, touch, light). Death is usually due to respiratory arrest.

Symptoms–Chronic: Not applicable.

Disease Confusion: Grand mal seizures, tetanus.

Victim Notes: Strychnine does not cause true seizures, and the patient is awake and painfully aware of the contractions.

DETECTION OF STRYCHNINE

Specimens: Food, beverages, medications, blood, urine, gastric contents, and autopsy organ specimens.

Method: Colorimetry, ultra-violet (UV) spectrophotometry, or gas chromatography (GC).

Toxic Levels:

Blood	Urine	Gastric	Other
21 mcg/mL	9.1 mcg/mL	61 mcg/mL	Unknown

SELECTED STRYCHNINE HOMICIDE CASES

Christina Edmunds (1871)

Thomas Cream (1892)

Jean-Pierre Vacquier (1924)

Ethel Major (1934)

Floyd Horton (1937)

Patsy Wright (1987)

THALLIUM

Form: Thallium in elemental form is a soft metal. Thallium can also exist as metallic salts (acetate, carbonate, chloride, sulfate, and so on).

Color: Thallium salts are white crystalline powders.

Odor: Odorless.

Solubility: Thallium salts are readily soluble in water.

Taste: Tasteless.

Source: Thallium can be used as a rodenticide and an insecticide, but the use is restricted to licensed applicators (public use prohibited since 1965). Thallium salts are widely used in industry (manufacture of optical lenses, photoelectric cells, costume jewelry) and chemical analyses.

Lethal Dose: Acute, 1 g, 12–15 mg/kg; Chronic, unknown.

How it Kills: Thallium causes membrane depolarization by acting as a substitute for potassium in the sodium-potassium-ATPase pump. Binds to enzymes containing (-SH) sulfhydral groups.

Poison Notes: Thallium is one of the most lethal poisons and produces one of the highest incidences of long-term sequellae (mainly neurological).

VICTIM OF THALLIUM

Administered: Can be given in food, drink, or medications.

Symptom Onset Time Interval: Thallium is rapidly absorbed through the skin, and mucous membranes of the mouth and GI tract. GI symptoms appear after a latent period of usually 12–24 hours.

Symptoms–Acute: Abdominal pain, anorexia, nausea, vomiting, diarrhea, delirium, depressed respirations, seizure, coma, and death.

Symptoms–Chronic: Muscle weakness, atrophy, tingling and numbness in the extremities, peripheral neuropathy, painful legs, feet feel like they are on fire, burning feeling in body, body sensitive to touch. Aldrich-Mees' lines (3–4 weeks post), hair loss (a classic symptom; may appear after 2–4 weeks).

Disease Confusion: Viral disease, Guillain-Barre syndrome.

Victim Notes: Victim is often misdiagnosed.

DETECTION OF THALLIUM

Specimens: Food, beverages, medications, saliva, blood, urine, gastric contents, hair, and autopsy organ specimens.

Method: Flameless atomic absorption.

Toxic Levels:

Blood	Urine	Gastric	Other
0.5–11 mg/L	1.7–11 mg/L	Unknown	Unknown

Analysis Notes: Because thallium is not a normal body constituent, any concentration is considered significant. Blood and hair thallium levels are not reliable measures of exposure.

SELECTED THALLIUM HOMICIDE CASES

Martha Lowenstein Marek (1932)

Caroline Grills (1947)

Graham Frederick Young (1971)

George Hanei (1976)

George Trepal (1988)

REFERENCES

Ballantyne B, Marrs TC (eds.): *Clinical and Experimental Toxicology of Cyanides,* Wright Publishers, Bristol, UK, 1987.

Baselt RC, Cravey RH: *Disposition of Toxic Drugs and Chemicals in Man,* 3rd ed. Year Book Medical Publishers, Inc., Chicago IL, 1989.

Bryson PD: *Comprehensive Review in Toxicology,* 2nd ed. Aspen Publishers, Inc., Rockville MD, 1989.

Ellenhorn MJ, Barceloux DG: *Medical Toxicology: Diagnosis and Treatment of Human Poisoning.* Elsevier, New York, NY, 1988.

Moyer TP: Heavy metals: the forgotten toxins. *Therapeutic Drug Monitoring and Clinical Toxicology Division,* July 1996; 11(3):1–5.

Olson KR: *Poisoning and Drug Overdose.* Appleton and Lange, Norwalk CT, 1990.

Polson CJ, Green MA, Lee MR: Clinical Toxicology, 3rd ed., J. B. Lippincott Co., Philadelphia, 1983.

Proctor NH, Hughes JP, Fischman ML: *Chemical Hazards of the Workplace*, 2nd ed. J. B. Lippincott Co., Philadelphia, 1988.

Seiler HG, Sigel H, Sigel A: *Handbook on Toxicity of Inorganic Compounds.* Marcel Dekker, Inc., New York, NY, 1988.

Bibliographies

This bibliography on forensic toxicology, poisoning murders, and poisons in general, represents the results of over 30 years of the author's research on the subject. The citations have been drawn from an in-depth review of the international literature. This extensive bibliography is included for two major purposes: (1) for those individuals wishing to study the subject of poisons and murder in even greater depth, these citations will serve as a catalogue of available literature, and (2) for criminal investigators, these bibliographies can serve as a checklist of published items for which to search in the environment of the homicidal poisoner.

POISONERS THROUGHOUT HISTORY

Adam HL: Pritchard the Poisoner. Mellifont Press, (no date)
Adams F: Remarks on the ancient principles of toxicology. *Edinburgh Med Surg J* 1830;33:315-333.
Addington A: *Trial of Mary Blandy*, Hodge, London, 1914.
Alamigeon F: Les experts medicaux du XIXe siecle confrontes aux empoisonnements criminels par l'arsenic (The medical experts of the 19th Century confront the criminal poisonings by arsenic). *Medical Thesis*, 1980, No. 555. (in French).
Altick RD: *Victorian Studies in Scarlet: Murders and Manners in the Age of Victoria.* W. W. Norton & Company, Inc., New York, NY, 1970.
Alvisi E: Cesare Borgia. Tip d'Ignazio Galeati e Figilo, Imola, Italy, 1878 (in Italian).
Ambelain R: *La chapelle des damnes: 1650–1703, la veritable Affaire des poisons*. R. Laffont, Paris, 1983 (in French).
Amos A: The Great Oyer of Poisoning: *The Trial of the Earl of Somerset for the Poisoning of Sir Thomas Overbury in the Tower of London and Various Matters Connected Therewith, From Contemporary Mss.* Richard Bentley, London, 1846.
Anonymous: *A Complete Report of the Trial of Dr. E. W. Pritchard, for the Alleged Poisoning of His Wife and Mother-in-Law*, William Kay, Edinburgh, Scotland, 1865.
Anderson C: *Bodies of Evidence: The True Story of Judias Buenoano, Florida's Serial Murderess.* Carol Publishing Group, Secaucus, NJ, 1991.
Anonymous: Poisons and poisoners: old and new. *Practitioner.* 1900;65:171–177.
Anonymous: *The Poison Fiend! Life, Crimes, and Conviction of Lydia Sherman, (the Modern Lucretia Borgia), Recently Tried in New Haven, CT.* Barclay & Co., Philadelphia, 1873.
Anspacher C: *The Trial of Dr. DeKaplany.* Frederick Fell, 1965.
Appleton A: *Mary Ann Cotton, Her Story and Trial.* Michael Joseph, 1973.
Arehart-Treichel J: *Poisons and Toxins.* Holiday House, New York, NY, 1976.
Armstrong MH: Medicine, murder and man. *Med-Legal J* 1964;32:28–39.
Bardens D: *The Ladykiller.* Peter Davies, 1972. (Discussion of the Landru case.)
Barfield V: *Woman on Death Row.* Oliver-Nelson, Nashville, TN., 1985.
Barker D: *Palmer: The Rugeley Poisoner.* Duckworth, London, 1935.
Barnes DN, Hevenor WS: *Trial of John Hendrickson Jr. for the Murder of his Wife Maria, by Poisoning...* Barnes & Hevenor, Albany, NY, 1853.
Barnesby N: *Illustrated Life and Career of William Palmer, of Rugeley.* Ward & Lock, London, 1856.
Barnesby N: *Illustrated and Unabridged Edition of the Times Report of the Trial of William Palmer for the Poisoning of John Parsons Cook at Rugeley, from the Short-Hand Notes Taken in the Central Criminal Court from Day to Day.* Ward & Lock, London, 1856.
Baron JH: Paintress, princess and physician's paramour: poison or perforation? *J Royal Soc Med*, 1998;1:213–216.
Barrowcliff D: The Stoneleigh abbey poisoning case. *Med Legal J* 1971;39(3):79–90.

Bartrip PWJ: How green was my valence? Environmental arsenic poisoning and the Victorian domestic ideal. *English Hist Rev* 1994;109(433):891.
Baslez L: *Poisons in Egyptian Antiquity.* E. Le Francois, Paris, 1933 (in French).
Beal E: *The Trial of Adelaide Bartlett for Murder.* Stevens & Haynes, London, 1886.
Bedford S: *The Trial of Dr. Adams.* Simon & Schuster, New York, NY, 1959.
Belle or the Ballad of Dr. Crippen. A program from a music hall musical performed at the Strand Theater, London, May 4, 1961. (Note: Considered by many to be in poor taste, it closed after a run of only six weeks.)
Bell M: *The Life and Times of Lucrezia Borgia.* Harcourt Brace, New York, NY, 1953.
Benezech M: Introduction a l'etude medico-psychologique de Marie Besnard (Introduction to the medico-psychological study of Marie Besnard). *Ann Med Psychol* 1985;143(5):409–448 (in French).
Benezech M, Pellet C: Trois empoisonnements devant les Assies de la Gironde au XXe siecle, ou les experts, l'arsenic et les vieilles dentelles (Three poisonings in front of the Assizes of the Gironde in the 20th Century, or the experts, of the arsenic and the ancient lace). *Bordeaux Med* 1984;17:13–21 (in French).
Bereanau V, Todorov K: *The Umbrella Murder.* Pendragon Press, Cambridge, UK, 1994. (Discussion of the Georgi Markov assassination case.)
Berence F: *Les Borgias.* Pierre Aliffe, Paris, 1966 (in French).
Besnard M: *The Trial of Marie Besnard.* Heinemann, London, 1963.
Black L: *The Prince of Poisoners.* Dial Press, New York, NY, 1932. (A fictionalized account of poisoner Thomas Griffiths Wainewright.)
Bernadac C: *Devil's Doctors: Medical Experiments on Human Subjects in the Concentration Camps.* Ferni Publishing House, Geneva, Switzerland, 1978.
Blackburn DJ: Human Harvest: *The Sacramento Murder Story.* Knightsbridge, New York, NY, 1990. (A discussion of the Dorothea Puente case.)
Bloom U: *The Girl Who Loved Crippen.* Hutchinson, London, 1957. (A novel based on the Crippen murder case.)
Blyth H: *Madeleine Smith.* Duckworth, London, 1975.
Bombaugh CC: Female poisoners, ancient and modern. *Johns Hopkins Hosp Bull* 1899;10:148–153.
Borowitz A: *Innocence and Arsenic: Studies in Crime and Literature.* Harper and Row, New York, NY, 1977.
Borowitz A: The Crippen scandal. *Cleveland Magazine,* January 1985;120–133.
Brackett DW: *Holy Terror: Armageddon in Tokyo.* Weatherhill. Inc., New York, NY, 1996.(A discussion of the nerve gas attack on the Tokyo subway in 1995).
Bradford S: *Cesare Borgia.* Macmillan, New York, NY, 1976.
Bradshaw JS: *Doctors on Trial.* Paddington Press, New York, NY, 1978.
Brenner J: *L'armorie aux poisons.* Grasset, Paris, 1976. (in French).
Bridges Y: *Poison and Adelaide Bartlett: The Pimlico Poisoning Case.* Macmillan, London, 1970. (A reissue of the 1962 work.)
Bridges Y: *How Charles Bravo Died: The Chronicles of a Cause Celebre.* Macmillan, London, 1970.
Brookes CJR: *Murder in Fact and Fiction.* Hurst and Blackett, London, 1926.
Brouardel P: *Les Empoisonnements* (The Poisonings). Baillere, Paris, 1902. (in French).

Brouardel P: *Les Intoxications* (The Intoxications). Baillere, Paris, 1904. (in French).
Brown W: *Introduction to Murder: The Unpublished Facts Behind the Lonelyhearts Killers, Martha Beck and Raymond Fernandez.* Greenberg, New York, NY, 1952.
Browne GL, Stewart CG: *Reports of Murder by Poisoning.* Steven & Sons, London, 1881.
Browne GL, Stewart CG: *Reports of Trials for Murder by Poisoning; by Prussic Acid, Strychnia, Antimony, Arsenic, and Aconita. Including the Trials of Tawell, W. Palmer, Dove, Madeline Smith, Dr. Pritchard, Smethurst, and Dr. Lamson.* Stevens & Sons, London, 1883.
Buchanan AJ: *The Trial of Ronald Geeves Griggs.* Famous Australian Trials, The Law Book Company of Australia, Sydney, Australia, 1930.
Budge EAW: *Amulets and Talismans.* University Books, New Hyde Park, NY, 1961.
Butler GL: *Madelaine Smith: Poisoner?* Duckworth, London, 1935.
Cabanes A, Nass L: *Poisons et sortileges. Les Cesars, envouteurs et sorciers, les Borgia...* (Poisons and spells. The Caesars, bewitchers and sorcerers, the Borgias), 1st series. Librarairie Plon, Paris, 1903 (in French).
Cabanes A, Nass L: *Poisons et sortileges. Les Medicis, les Bourbons, la Science au XXe Siecle,* (Poisons and spells. The Medicis, the Bourbons, the Science in the 20th Century), 2nd series. Librarairie Plon, Paris, 1903 (in French).
Cameron JM, Hardy AJ: The Brighton poisoning case 1872. *Practitioner,* 1972;208:401–405.
Camp J: *One Hundred Years of Medical Murder.* Bodley Head, UK, 1982. (Discussions of Palmer, Smethurst, Pritchard, Lamson, and Cream cases.)
Capp B: Serial killers in 17th-century England. *History Today* 1996;46(3):21–26.
Cashman J: *The Gentleman from Chicago: Being an Account of the Doings of Thomas Neill Cream, M.D. (M'Gill), 1850–1892.* Harper and Row, New York, NY, 1973. (A fictional work based on the activities of the real poisoner Thomas Neill Cream, MD.)
Cher M: *Poison at Court: Certain Figures of the Reign of Louis the Fourteenth.* D. Appleton, New York, NY, 1931.
Christie TL: *Etched in Arsenic: A New Study of the Maybrick Case.* JB Lippincott, Philadelphia, 1968.
Clarkson W: *Doctor's of Death: Ten True Stories of Doctors Who Kill.* Barricade Books, Fort Lee, NJ, 1992. (Rather sensational discussions about the following physician poisoners: Carl Coppolino, Paul Vickers, Geza DeKaplany, Henry Sugar, and Sam Dubria.)
Clarkson W: *Love You to Death, Darling: Murderous Wives.* Blake, 1992.
Collison–Morley L: *The Story of the Borgias.* Routledge, London, 1932.
Constantine-Quinn M: *Doctor Crippen.* The Rogue's Gallery, Duckworth, London, 1935.
Cook TH: *Early Graves: A Shocking True–Crime Story of the Youngest Woman Ever Sentenced to Death Row.* Dutton, New York, NY, 1990. (A discussion of the Judith Ann Neelley case.)
Coppolino CA: *The Crime That Never Was.* Justice Press, Tampa, FL, 1980.
Cornu M: *Le proces de la Marquise de Brinvilliers* (The legal action of the Marquise of Brinvilliers). Paris, 1894. (in French).

Costello LS: *The Queen's Poisoner or France in the Sixteenth Century.* R. Bentley, London, England, 1841. (3 vols; deals with Marguerite de Navarre, Rochellois, Catherine of Condi, etc., concerning the courts of Charles IX, and Henry III.)
Coulas I: The Borgias. Barnes & Noble Books, New York, NY, 1993.
Cowan H: *Report of the Trial of John Thompson Alias Peter Walker...For The Murder of Agnes Montgomery By Prussic Acid.* Thomas Constable, Edinburgh, Scotland, 1858.
Crimes of Passion. Treasure Press, London, 1983.
Cromie R, Wilson T: *The Romance of Poisons Being Weird Episodes from Life.* Jarrold and Sons, London, 1903.
Crompton R: Georgi Markov: death in a pellet, *Med-Legal J*, 1980;48(2):51–62.
Cullen T: *The Mild Murderer: The True Story of the Dr. Crippen Case.* Houghton Mifflin, New York, NY, 1977.
Cumston CG: The victim of the Medicis and the Borgias in France from a medical standpoint. *Albany M Ann*, 1906;27:567–590.
Cumston, CG: XVI poisoning cases aspects. *Med-Legal J*, 1905;23–172.
Davies E: Popular errors about poisons: uncanny examples of poisoning, both attempted and accomplished in the 18th and 19th centuries. *Proceedings of the Literary and Philosophical Society of Liverpool*, 66th Session, 1876–77; 229–244.
Davies N: *Murder on Ward Four.* Chatto and Windus, England, 1993, (A discussion of the Beverly Allitt case.)
Davis EW: The ethnobiology of the Haitian zombi. *J Ethnopharmacol*, 1983;9:85–104.
Davis EW: Preparation of the Haitian zombi poison. *Botanical Museum Leaflets*, Harvard University press, Cambridge, MA, 1983;29(2):139–149.
Davis EW: *The Serpent & the Rainbow: A Harvard Scientist's Astounding Journey into the Secret Societies of Haitian Voodoo, Zombies and Magic.* Simon and Schuster, New York, NY, 1985.
Davison A: Murder and medicine. *Report Proc Scottish Society History Med*, 1969;15–27.
Decourt P: L'affaire LaFarge: histoire d'un crime judiciaire (The LaFarge case: history of a legal crime). *Archives Internationales Claude Bernard*, 1974;2(5):155–206 (in French).
DeFord MA: *The Overbury Affair.* Chilton Co., Philadelphia, PA, 1960.
De La Torre L: *The Truth About Belle Gunness.* Fawcett, New York, NY, 1955.
De Pasquale A: Pharmacognosy: the oldest modern science. *J Ethnopharmacol*, 1984;11:1–16.
Desmaze C: *Histoire de la medicine legale en France d'Apres les Lois, registres et arrets criminels.* Paris, 1880, (in French).
Devlin P: *Easing the Passing: The Trial of Dr. John Bodkin Adams.* Bodley Head, London, 1985.
Dew W: *I Caught Crippen: Memoirs of Ex-Chief Inspector Walter Dew.* Blackie & Son, London, 1938.
Dewes S: *Doctors of Murder.* John Long, London, 1962.
Doremus RO, Witthaus RA: *Chemistry of the Cobb-Bishop Poisoning.* New York, NY, 1879.

Dornhorst P: *They Fly by Twilight: A Play in Three Acts.* Thomas Nelson, London, 1940. (A play based upon the Crippen case, first performed in 1938.)

Dragstedt CA: Trial by ordeal. *Quart Bull Northwestern Univ Med School,* 1945; 19:136–141.

Dupre E: History of poisoning. *Arch Anthropol Crim,* 1909;24:5.

Eaton H: *Famous Poison Trials.* W. Collins Sons & Co. Ltd., London, 1923. (Discussions about the following poisoners: Aconitine [Lamson], Antimony [Pritchard], Arsenic [Seddon], Hyoscine [Crippen], and Strychnine (Palmer)).

Eckert WG: Historical aspects of poisoning and toxicology. *Amer J Foren Med Pathol,* 1980;1(3):261–264.

Eckert WG: Physician crimes and criminals: the historical and forensic aspects. *Amer J Foren Med Pathol,* 1982; 3(1):221–230.

Eckert WG: The development of forensic medicine in the United Kingdom from the 18th century. *Am J Foren Med Pathol,* 1992;13(2):124–131.

Elkind P: *The Death Shift: The True Story of Nurse Genene Jones and the Texas Baby Murders.* Viking Press, New York, NY, 1989.

Erlanger R: *Lucrezia Borgia: A Biography.* Dutton, New York, NY, 1978.

Etiemble: *Mes contre-poisons.* Gallimard, Paris, 1974 (in French).

Everitt D: *Human Monsters: An Illustrated Encyclopedia of the World's Most Vicious Murderers.* Contemporary Books, Chicago, IL, 1993.

Farrell M: *Poisons and Poisoners: An Encyclopedia of Homicidal Poisonings.* Robert Hale, London, 1992.

Ferrara O: *The Borgia Pope.* Sheed and Ward, New York, NY,1940.

Fido M: *Murder Guide to London.* Academy of Chicago Publishers, Chicago, IL, 1990.

Fletcher G: *The Life and Career of Dr. William Palmer of Rugeley: Together with a Full Account of the Murder of John P. Cook and A Short Account of his Trial in May 1856.* T. Fisher Unwin, London, 1925.

Forshufvud S: *Napoleon a-t-il ete Empoisonne.* Plon, Paris, 1961 (in French).

Forshufvud S, Smith H, Wassen A: Arsenic content of Napoleon I's hair probably taken immediately after his death. *Nature,* 1961;4789:103–105.

Franke D: *The Torture Doctor.* Hawthorne Books, New York, NY, 1975. (A discussion of the case of Herman W. Mudgett, *alias* Henry H. Holmes.)

Frasier DK: *Murder Cases of the Twentieth Century: Biographies and Bibliographies of 280 Convicted or Accused Killers.* McFarland, Jefferson, NC.

Full Report, of the Extraordinary and Interesting Trial of Miss Madeleine Smith...on the Charge of Poisoning by Arsenic Her Late Lover, 5th ed. Read, London, 1857.

Funk-Bretano F: *Le drame des poisons* (The poison drama). Hachette, Paris, 1909 (in French). (Chapters include: Marie-Madeleine of Brinvilliers, The Drama of Poisons in the Court of Louis LIV, The Death of "Madame," Root of the Affair of Poisons, and The Fortune-Teller.)

Funk-Bretano F: *Princes and Poisoners.* Duckworth, London, 1901.

Funk-Bretano F: *Lucrece Borgia.* La Nouvelle Revu Critique, 1930.

Furneaux R: *The Medical Murderer.* Abelard-Schuman, New York, NY, 1957. (Discussions about the following poisoners: Palmer, Smethurst, Lamson, Cream, Pritchard, and Crippen.)

Fusero C: *The Borgias*. (Trans. Peter Green.) Frederick A. Praeger, New York, NY, 1972.
Gaute JHH, Odell R: *The Murderers' Who's Who.* Harrap Ltd., London, 1982.
Gaute JHH, Odell R: *Murder Whatdunit.* Harrap Ltd., London, 1982.
Gaute JHH, Odell R: *Murder Whereabouts.* Harrap Ltd., London, 1986.
Gaute JHH, Odell R: *The New Murderer's Who's Who.* Dorset, UK, 1991. (A completely revised and updated edition.)
Gee D: *Poison: The Coward's Weapon.* Whitcoulls Publishers, Christchurch, New Zealand, 1985. (A collection of New Zealand poisoning crime cases from 1859 onward.)
Gemelli P: *Les poisons de Beaubourg, ou L'affaire Lamotte.* Denoel, Paris, 1987. (in French).
Gettler AO: The historical development of toxicology: with interesting cases from the files of the chief medical examiner's office of New York City. *J Foren Sci* 1956;1:3–25.
Gilbert M: Dr. *Crippen* Famous Criminal Trials Series, Odhams Press, London, 1953.
Gilbert W: *Lucrezia Borgia*. Hurst and Blackett, London, 1864.
Gimlette JD: *Malay Poisons and Charm Cures.* J & A Churchill, London, 1923.
Ginsburg P: *Poisoned Blood: A True Story of Murder, Passion, and an Astonishing Hoax.* Scribner's, New York, NY, 1975. (A discussion of the Marie Hilley Case of poisoning with arsenic.)
Glaister J: *The Power of Poison*. William Morrow, New York, NY, 1954.
Good J, Goreck S: *Poison Mind: The True Story of the Mensa Murderer and the Policewoman Who Risked Her Life to Bring Him to Justice,* William Morrow, New York, NY, 1995. (A discussion of the George Trepal case of poisoning with thallium.)
Goodman J: *The Crippen File.* Allison & Busby, London, 1985.
Goodman J: *Medical Murders.* Carol Publishing Group, New York, NY, 1992. (A discussion of: Lamson, Palmer, Smethurst, Waite, Cream, Petiot, Pritchard, and Waddingham.)
Goodman J: *Acts of Murder: True-life Murder Cases from the World of Stage and Screen.* Carol Publishing Group, Secaucus, NJ, 1993.
Goodman R: *The Private Life of Dr. Crippen: A Novel.* Heinemann, London, 1981. (A fictional account of the Crippen case.)
Gordeux P: *Le Docteur Petiot.* Editions j'ai lu, Paris, 1970 (in French).
Gordon A: *The Lives of Pope Alexander VI and his Son Caesar Borgia* C. Davis & T. Green, London, 1929 (2 vols).
Gordon R: *The Private Life of Doctor Crippen.* Heinemann, 1981.
Graves R: *They Hanged My Saintly Billy: the Life and Death of Dr. William Palmer.* Doubleday, New York, NY, 1957.
Griffiths A: The poisoners, In: *Mysteries of Police and Crime,* Cassell, London, 1890, 14–89 (3 vols).
Gril E: *Madame LaFarge devant ses juges.* Gallimard, Paris, 1958 (in French).
Grim-Samuel V: On the mushroom that defied the Emperor Claudius. *Classical Quart*. 1991;41:178–182.

Grombach JV: *The Great Liquidator.* Doubleday, New York, NY, 1980. (A discussion of the Marcel Petiot case.)

Gwynm G: *Did Adelaide Bartlett, Administer the Chloroform...?* Johnson, 1950.

Gyorfyey F: Arsenic and no lace. *Caduceus,* 1987;3(2):40–65. (A discussion of the mass arsenic poisonings in Nagyrev, Hungary.)

Haines M: *Doctors Who Kill.* Toronto Sun Publishers, Toronto, Canada, 1993.

Hall J: *The Bravo Mystery and Other Cases.* Bodley Head, London, 1923.

Hall J (ed.): *The Trial of Adelaide Bartlett.* Wm. Hodge & Co., England, 1927.

Hallworth R, Williams M: *Where There's a Will: The Sensational Life of Dr. John Bodkin Adams.* The Capstans Press, Jersey, UK, 1983.

Hardwick M: *Doctors on Trial.* Jenkins, 1961.

Harter K: *Winter of Frozen Dreams.* Contemporary Books, Chicago, IL, 1990. (A discussion of the Barbara Hoffman case.)

Hartman MS: *Victorian Murderesses: A True History of Thirteen Respectable French and English Women Accused of Unspeakable Crimes.* Schoken Books, New York, NY, 1977. (Discussions about the following poisoners: Adelaide Bartlett, Florence Bravo, Euphemie Lacoste, Marie LaFarge, Florence Maybrick, and Madeleine Smith.)

Harris SH: *Factories of Death: Japanese Biological Warfare, 1932–45, and the American Cover-Up.* Routledge, New York, NY, 1995.

Hefland WH: The poisoning of the sick at Jaffa, *Veroffenthichun des Internationalen Gesellschaft fur Gershichte der Pharmazie,* 1975;42:79–97.

Hemming R: *With Murderous Intent.* Onyx, New York, NY, 1991. (A discussion of the David Richard Davis case.)

Heppenstall R: *Bluebeard and After: Three Decades of Murder in France.* Peter Owen, London, 1972.

Hervey C: Report on the crime of thuggee by means of poisons in British territory for the years 1864, 1865, and 1866. General Superintendents's Office, Delhi, India, 1868.

Hillairet JB: *Historic Notes on Arsenic Poisoning.* A. Bailly, Paris, 1847.

The History of the Most Remarkable Tryals in Great Britain and Ireland, in Capital Cases. A. Bell, London, 1715 (2 vols.)

Ho PY: Elixir poisoning in China—medieval. *Janus,* 1959;48(4):221.

Hoffman RH, Bishop J: *The Girl in Poison Cottage.* Gold Medal, 1953.

Holden A: *The St. Albans Posoner: The life and crimes of Graham Young,* Hodder & Stoughton, London, 1974. (Republished in 1995, by Corgi Books, UK.)

Holmes P: *The Trials of Dr. Coppolino.* New American Library, New York, NY, 1968.

Honeycombe G: *The Murders of the Black Museum: 1870–1970.* Hutchinson, London, 1982.

Honeycombe G: *More Murders of the Black Museum: 1835–1985.* Hutchinson, London, 1993.

Hoskins P: *Two Men Were Acquitted: The Trial and Acquittal of Doctor John Bodkin Adams.* Secker & Warburg, London, 1984.

Hsu Y: *History of Toxicology in China.* Hsin i shi-chu Co., Hangchow, 1955.

Hubert D: *Les hommes–poisons.* Hachette, Paris, 1970 (in French).
Hughes-Wilson J: Who killed Napoleon? An historic murder solved. *RUSI J* Dec. 1997;55–60.
Hunt P: *The Madeleine Smith Affair.* Carroll & Nicholson, London, 1950.
Illustrated Life and Career of William Palmer, of Rugeley: Containing Details of His Conduct as...Poisoner, with Original Letters...and Other Authenticated Documents. Ward and Lock, London, 1856.
Ingram D: *A Strict and Impartial Enquiry into the Cause and Death of the late William Scawen, Esq; in Surry, ascertaining, from the Medical Evidence against Jane Butterfield, the Impossibility of Poison having been given him. To which is added, An Account of Accidental Poisons, to which Families are Exposed, with their Antidotes, under...Stings and Bites, Vegetables, Minerals, Fumes and Vapours.* T. Cadell, London, 1777.
Irvine A, Johnson H: R vs Young: murder by thallium. *Medico-Legal J,* 42(3),1974,76–90.
Iung T: *La verite sur le masque fer (Les Empoisonneurs)* [The truth under the iron mask (The Poisoners]), Paris, France, 1873 (in French).
Jackman T, Troy C: *Rites of Burial.* Windsor, New York, NY, 1992. (A discussion of the Robert Berdella case.)
Janus: Aqua Tofana, 5, 27, 1900.
Jeffers HP: *Bloody Business: An Anecdotal History of Scotland Yard.* Pharos Books, New York, NY, 1992.
Jeffreys JG: *A Conspiracy of Poisons.* Walker, New York, NY, 1977.
Jensen LB: *Poisoning Misadventures.* Charles C. Thomas, Springfield, IL, 1977, pp. 112–116,158–164.
Jesse FT: *The Trial of Madeline Smith.* Day, New York, NY, 1927.
Johnson WB: *The Age of Arsenic: Being an Account of the Life, Trial, and Execution of Catherine Montvoison, known as La Voison, and of her vile Associates and credulous Clients of both high and low Degree: together with a Relation of their various Transactions in Poison, Abortion, and Black or Satanic Masses, with other Details concerning sundry Manners and Habits of the Times and with but little Moralizing thereon: the Whole comprising a curious and momentous episode in the Reign of King Louis XIV of France.* Jonathan Cape & Robert Ballou, New York, NY, 1932.
Jones A: *Women Who Kill.* Holt, Rinehart & Winston, New York, NY, 1981.
Jones DEH, Arsenic in Napoleon's wallpaper. *Nature,* 1982;299:626–627.
Jones RB: *Palmer The Rugeley Poisoner.* Daisy Bank Publications, UK ~1910.
Jones RG: *POISON! The World's Greatest True Murder Stories.* Lyle Stuart Inc., Secaucus, NJ, 1987.
Kaplan J, Papajohn G, Zorn E: *Murder of Innocence: The Tragic Life and Final Rampage of Laurie Dann.* Warner Books, 1990. (Discussion of the Laurie Dann case, who attempted in 1988, to poison 50 people on Chicago's North Shore.)
Katz L: *The Coppolino Murder Trial.* Bee-Line Books, New York, NY, 1967.
Kaufman DB: Poisons and poisonings among the Romans. *Classical Philology* 1932;27:156–167.
Kent A: *The Death Doctors.* New English Library, London, 1975.

Kent A: *Deadly Medicine: Doctors and True Crime.* Toplinger Pub. Co., New York, NY, 1975.

Kenyon FW: *The Naked Sword: The Story of Lucrezia Borgia.* Dodd Mead & Co., New York, NY, 1968.

Kershaw *A: Murder in France.* Constable & Comp. Ltd., London, 1955. (Discussions about the following poisoners: Girard, Petiot.)

Kinder G: *Victim, the Other Side of Murder.* Delacorte Press, New York, NY, 1982. (A discussion of the Dale Selby Pierre case.)

Kogon E: *Nazi Mass Murder: A Documentary History of the Use of Poison Gas.* Yale University Press, New Haven, CT, 1993.

Kohn GC: *Dictionary of Culprits and Criminals.* The Scarecrow Press, Inc., Metuchen, NY 1986.

Kozminska: A history of poisons and poisoners. *Arch Med Sad* 1955;7:113. (in Polish).

Lakie MH, Cook G, MacMurray D: A 17th century poisoning case. *Pharmaceuti Historian.* 6(2),1976.

Lane B: *The Murder Club: Guide to London.* Harrap Ltd., London, 1988. (Discussions about the following poisoners: GH Lamson, FH Seddon, HH Crippen, and the murder of Edwin Bartlett.)

Lane B: *The Murder Club: Guide to South-East England.* Harrap Ltd., London, 1988. (Discussions about the following poisoners: FG Radford, Percy Mapleton, murder of HG Chevis, and Jean-Pierre Vaquier.)

Lane B: *The Murder Club—Guide to North-West England.* Harrap Ltd., London, 1988. (Discussions about the following poisoners: Bingham Case, death of James Finlay, Charlie Parton, and Dr. R.G. Clements.)

Lane B: *The Murder Club—Guide to the Midlands.* Harrap Ltd., London, 1988. (discussions about the following poisoners: H.R. Armstrong, B.A. Pace, John Donellan, Dorothea Waddingham, and E.L. Major.)

Lane B: *The Murder Club—Guide to the Eastern and Home Counties.* Harrap Ltd., London, 1989. (Discussions about the following poisoners: Elizabeth Fenning, Amy Hutchinson, John Tawell, and Graham Young.)

Lane B: *The Murder Club—Guide to South-West England and Wales.* Harrap Ltd., London, 1989. (Discussion about the following poisoners: Edward Ernest Black, Mary Channel, Charlotte Bryant, Jane Cox, the murder of Mabel Greenwood, and the murder of Alice ["Annie"] Thomas.)

Langlois JL: *Belle Guness: The Lady Bluebeard.* Indiana University Press, Bloomington, IN, 1985.

Latour A: *The Borgias,* (trans. Neil Mann). Abelard-Schuman, New York, NY, 1963.

LaWall CH: *Four Thousand Years of Pharmacy.* J. B. Lippincott Comp., Philadelphia, PA, 1927,297–303.

Lebigre A: *L'affaire des poisons: 1679–1682.* Editions Complexe, Brussels, Belgium, 1989.

Legue G: *Medicine et empoisinnements au XVIIe siecle* (Medicine and Poisonings in the 17th century). Bibliotheque-Charpentier, Lyon, France, 1895 (in French).

Legue G: *Medecins et empoisonneurs au XVIIe siecle* (Medicines and Poisoners in the 17th Century). Paris, 1896. (in French) (Reprinted in 1903).

Legue G: *17th Century Poisoners.* Charpentier & Fasquelle, Paris, 1895 (in French).

Legue G: Women poisoners in history. *Med-Legal J* 1903;10:152.

Lemoine J: *Madame de Montespan et la legende des poisons* (Madame Montespan and the Legend of Poisons). Paris, 1908 (in French).

LeNeve *E: Ethel LeNeve: Her Life Story: With the True Account of Their Flight and Her Friendship for Dr. Crippen. Also Startling Particulars of Her Life at Hilldrop Cresent —Told by Herself.* Publishing Office, Haymarket, London, 1910. (This three-penny pamphlet, which was sold on the streets of England, was an illegally produced reproduction of accounts that were first published in the *Lloyd's Weekly News* of Nov. 6,13, 1910.)

Lepine P: Un dossier conteste: l'affaire LaFarge (A debatable record of the LaFarge matter). *Lyon Pharmaceutique,* 1980,31(1):39–44 (in French).

Levitt L: *The Healer: A True Story of Medicine and Murder.* Viking Press, New York, NY, 1980. (A discussion of the of the Dr. Charles Friedgood case.)

Levy JH: *The Necessity for Criminal Appeal as Illustrated by the Maybrick Case.* King, London, 1899.

Lewin L: *Die Gifte in der Weltgeschichte: Toxikologische, Algemein-Verstandliche Untersuchungen der Historischen Quellen* (Poisoning in World History). Verlag Von Julius Springer, Berlin, Germany, 1920 (in German).

Lewin PK: Napoleon Bonaparte: no evidence of chronic arsenic poisoning. *Nature* 1982;299:628–629.

Lewis RH: *Victorian Murders.* David & Charles, London, 1988. (Discussions of the following poisoners: William Palmer, MD, Adelaide Bartlett, Madeline Smith, Florence Maybrick, Edith Carew, Thomas Smethurst, MD, Mary Leffey, George Lamson, MD, J. Milton Bowers, MD, Edward Wm. Pritchard, MD, Carlyle Harris, Robert Buchanan, MD, Thomas Neill Cream, MD, and the murder of Charles Bravo.)

Lewis RH: *Edwardian Murders.* David & Charles, London, 1989. (Discussions of the following poisoners: Johann Hoch, George Chapman, Hawley Crippen, MD, Henri Girard, Arthur Waite DDS, Bennett Hyde MD, Richard Brinkley, Roland Molineux, Albert Patrick, and the murder of Henry Bingham.)

Linedecker CL, Burt WA: *Nurses Who Kill.* Pinnacle Books, Windsor Publishing Corp., New York, NY, 1990. (Discussions of the Richard Angelo, and Donald Harvey cases.)

Lloyd M: *The Guiness Book of Espionage.* Da Capo Press, New York, NY, 1994.

Lucas-Dubreton J: *The Borgias,* (trans. Philip John Stead). E.P. Dutton, New York, NY, 1956.

MacDonald JD: *No Deadly Drug.* Doubleday, 1968. New York, NY, (Discussion of the case of Dr. Carl Coppolino).

MacDougall AW: *The Maybrick Case: A Settlement of the Case As a Whole.* Baliere, Tindall & Cox, London, 1896.

Mackay C: The Slow Poisoners, In: *Extraordinary Popular Delusions and the Madness of Crowds.* Barnes and Noble, New York, NY, 1993;569–592. (A reprint of the 1852 edition.)

Mackenzie F: *Landru.* Charles Scribner's Sons, New York, NY, 1928.
MacNalty A: *The Princes in the Tower and Other Royal Mysteries.* 1955.
Maeder T: *The Unspeakable Crimes of Dr. Petiot.* Penguin Books, U K, 1980.
Maitai CK, Faure J, Yacoub M: A survey on the use of poisoned arrows in Kenya during the period 1964–1971, *East Afr Med J* 1973;50(2):100–104.
Mallet ME: *The Borgias.* Bodley Head, London, 1969.
Mathew AH: *The Life and Times of Rodrigo Borgia.* St. Paul, London, 1912.
Mandelsberg RG: *Medical Murderers.* Pinnacle Books, Windsor Publishing Corp., New York, NY, 1992.
Mandin L: *Racine, le Sadisme et l'affaire des poisons Mercure de France.* France, 1940 (in French).
Mann J: *Murder, Magic, and Medicine.* Oxford University Press, New York, NY, 1993.
Marriner B: *Murder With Venom.* True Crime Library, No. 4, Forum Press, London, 1993.
Martinetz D, Lohs K: *Poison: Sorcery and Science—Friend and Foe.* Grafische Werke Zwickau, Leipzig, Germany, 1987. (Translated from the German by Alistair and Alison Wightman.)
Massengill SE: *A Sketch of Medicine and Pharmacy.* S.E. Massengill Company, Bristol, TN, 1942, 311–361.
Masson A: *La Sorcellerie et la Science des Poisons au XVII Siecle* (Witchcraft and Poisoning of the 17th Century). Librarie Hachette, Paris, 1904 (in French).
Masson R: *Number One: A Story of Landru* (trans. Gillian Tindall). Hutchinson, London, 1964.
Massu GV: *L'Enquete Petiot* (The Petiot Inquiry). Librarie Artheme Fayard, Paris, 1959 (in French).
Mattossian MK: *Poisons of the Past: Molds, Epidemics and History.* Yale University Press, New Haven, CT, 1989.
Maybrick F: *Mrs. Maybrick's Own Story: My 15 Lost Years.* Funk & Wagnall, New York, NY, 1905.
McDonald RR: *Black Widow: The True Story of the Hilley Poisonings.* New Horizon Press, New York, NY, 1986 (a discussion of the Marie Hilley case.)
McElwe E: *The Murder of Sir Thomas Overbury.* New York, NY, 1952.
McLaren A: *A Prescription for Murder: The Victorian Serial Killings of Dr. Thomas Neill Cream.* University of Chicago Press, Chicago, IL, 1993.
Meadley R: *Classics in Murder: True Stories of Infamous Crimes as Told by Famous Crime Writers.* Ungar Publishing, New York, NY, 1986. (Discussions of the following poisoners: Dr. Crippen, and Mary Blandy)
Meadows C: *Henbane.* V. Gollancz, London, 1935. (A novel based on the Crippen case, published in the USA as *Doctor Moon*, G.B. Putnam's Sons, 1935.)
Meek WJ: The gentle art of poisoning (reprinted from *Phi Beta Pi Quarterly*, May 1928). *Medico-Historical Papers*, University of Wisconsin, Madison, WI, 1954,pp. 1–11.
Micca G: Historic poisons and poisoning. *Minerva Med* 1968;59:5015.
Milt B: 1737 Poison Case in Zurich. *Gesneurs (Aarau)* 1953;10(1/2):79.
Moncel C: Baudliere, les poisons et l'inconnu: essai. Riorges, Moncel, 1974.

Mongredien G: *Madame de Montespan et l'affaire des poisons* (Madame Montespan and the Affair of Poisons). Paris, 1953 (in French).

Montespan M: *Memoirs of Madame la Marquise de Montespan* (trans. P.E.P.). Grover Society, London, 1904.

Moore K, Reed D: *Deadly Medicine: The Chilling True Story of a Pediatric Nurse Who Murdered Scores of Her Infant Patients.* St. Martin's Press, New York, NY, 1988. (A discussion of the Genene Jones case.)

Morison J: *A Complete Report of the Trial of Miss Madeleine Smith.* Wm. P. Nimmo, Edinburgh, Scotland, 1857.

Morland S: *That Nice Miss Smith,* St. Martin's Press, New York, NY, 1988.

Morrison JTJ: *Poisons.* Benn, London, 1930.

Mortimer J: *Famous Trials.* Dorset Press, New York, NY, 1984. (Discussions of the following poisoners: Madeleine Smith, Dr. Crippen, and H.R. Armstrong)

Mossiker F: *The Affair of the Poisons: Louis XIV, Madame de Montespan and One of History's Great Unsolved Mysteries.* Alfred A. Knopf, New York, NY, 1969.

Muntner S: *Treatise on Poisons and their Antidotes, (The Medical Writings of Moses Maimonides vol. 2).* Lippincott & Co., Montreal, Canada, 1966.

Murder Casebook, a magazine series, by Marshall Cavendish Ltd., London, 1989–1993.

9 - *The Mild-Mannered Murderer*: HH Crippen Case.
#40 - *Eastbourne's Doctor Death*: Bodkin Adams Case.
#41 - *The Poisoners:* Florence Maybrick, and Henry Seddon Cases.
#50 - *France's Angel of Death*: Marcel Petiot Case.
#53 - *The Croydon Poisonings*: Grace Duff Case.
#57 - *The Modern Bluebeard*: Henri Landru Case.
#59 - *A Passion for Poisoning*: Graham Young Case.
#65 - *Adultery and Arsenic*: H.R. Armstrong, Greenwood, and Arthur Waite Cases.
#85 - *She-Devil:* Simone Weber Case.
#94 - *The Whisperings*: Marie Besnard, and Louisa Merrifield Cases.
#105 - *A Woman's Weapon*: Charlotte Bryant, Ethel Major, and Violette Nozieres Cases.
#107 - *Traces of Poison*: Florence Bravo, and Adelaide Bartlett Cases.
#118 - *Imperfect Parents*: Marie Hilley Case.
#122 - *Deadly Doctors*: Carl Coppolino, and Geza DeKaplany Cases.

Murgatroyd E: *Cooking to Kill! The Poison Cook-book: Comic Recipes for the Ghoul, Cannibal, Witch & Murderer. Stewing and potting mothers-in-law. Tested recipes for spoiled brats, business rivals, and strayed lovers. Cannibal picnic meat. Sure-fire salads. How to make friends die laughing.* Peter Pauper Press, Mount Vernon, NY, 1951. (A humorous book discussing poison recipes.)

Nash JR: *Look for the Woman: A Narrative Encyclopedia of Female Poisoners. Kidnappers, Thieves, Extortionists, Terrorists, Swindlers and Spies from Elizabethan Times to the Present.* M. Evans, New York, NY, 1981.

Nash JR: *Encyclopedia of World Crime,* (6 volumes) Crime Books, Inc., Wilmette, Ill., 1990. (contains over 10,000 criminal biographical sketches, including over 300 poisoners!)

Nass L: Les empoisonnements sous Louis XIV (Poisonings under Louis XIV). Carre et Naud, *These Med*, Paris, 1898 (in French).
Neville R, Clarke J: *The Life and Crimes of Charles Sobhraj*. J. Cape, London, 1979.
Nezondet R: *Petiot "le possede"*. Paris,1950 (in French).
Norman C: *The Genteel Murderer*. Macmillan, New York, NY, 1956. (The life of Thomas Griffiths Wainewright.)
Notable British Trial Series. W. Hodge, UK.
Trial of H.R. Armstrong, ed. by Filson Young.
Trial of Adelaide Bartlett, ed. by Sir John Hall.
Trial of George Chapman, ed. by H.L. Adam, 1930.
Trial of Neill Cream, ed. by W. Teignmouth Shore, 1923.
Trial of H.H. Crippen, ed. by Filson Young, 1920.
Trial of Harold Greenwood, ed. by Winifred Duke, 1930.
Trial of Dr. Lamson, ed. by H.L. Adam, 1913.
Trial of Mrs. Maybrick, ed by H.B. Irving, 1912.
Trial of William Palmer, ed. by G.H. Knott, 1912.
Trial of Dr. Pritchard, ed. by Wm. Roughead, 1906.
Trial of The Seddons, ed. by Filson Young, 1914.
Trial of Madelaine Smith, ed. by A. Duncon Smith, 1905.
Trial of Madelaine Smith, ed. by F. Tennyson Jesse, 1927.
Norton C: *Disturbed Ground: The True Story of a Diabolical Female Serial Killer*. W. Morrow, New York, NY, 1994. (A discussion of the Dorothea Puente case)
Ober WB: Did Socrates die of hemlock poisoning? *New York State J Med*, 1977;77(2):254-258.
Odell R: *Exhumation of a Murder: The Crimes, Trial and Execution of a Perfect English Gentleman*. Proteus, London, 1978. (Discussion of the case of Major Herbert Rowse Armstrong.)
Odell R: *Exhumation of a Murder: The Life and Trial of Major Armstrong*. Harrap, London, 1975.
Odell R: *Landmarks In 20th Century Murder*. Headline Book Publishers, London, 1995.
Oehme P: History: poison deaths up to 20th century. *A Aerztl Fortbild (Jena)* 1965;59:278.
Olsen G: *Bitter Almonds: The True Story of Mothers, Daughters, and the Seattle Cyanide Murders*. Warner Books, New York, NY, 1993. (A discussion of the Stella Nickell case.)
Osius TG: The historic art of poisoning. *Univ Michigan Med Bull* 1957;23(3):111–116.
Paddock FK, Loomis CC, Perkons AK: An inquest on the death of Charles Francis Hall. *NEJM* 1970;282(14):784–786.
Palmer H; Dr. Adams' Trial for Murder. *Criminal Law Rev*, 1957;365–377.
Parry EA: *The Overbury Mystery*. Unwin, London, 1925.
Parry LA: *Some Famous Medical Trials*. Churchill, London, 1927.
Parry LA (ed.): *Trial of Dr. Smethurst*. Canada Law Book Co., Toronto, Canada, 1931.
Pejsa J: *The Molineux Affair*. St. Martin's Press, New York, NY, 1987.
Penzer NM: *Poison–Damsels and Other Essays in Folklore and Anthropology*. privately published, London, 1952.

Perry J, Chabert J: *L'affaire Petiot*. Gallimard, Paris, 1957. (In French).
Petifils JC: *L'affaire des poisons: alchimistes et sorciers sous Louis XIV*. A. Michel, Paris, 1977. (in French).
Piga A: Criminal poisoning: historical to 1940. *Forenses (Madr.)* 1946;3(58):1, (Continued in *Rev Med Leg (Madr)*, 1946;1(6):5.)
Piga A: History of Borgias: poisoners. *Rev Med Leg (Madr)* 1959;14:154.
Piper L: *Murder by Gaslight*. Gallery, New York, NY, 1991.
Pirot E: *La Marquis de Brinvilliers, recit de ses derniers moments* (The Marquis of Brinvilliers, an account of her final moments). Paris, 1883. (in French).
Plaidy J: *A Triptych of Poisoners.* Barnes & Noble Books, New York, NY, 1994. (Discussions on Cesare Borgia, La Marquise de Brinvilliers, and Dr. Edward Pritchard.)
Poison at the Priory, The Sunday Times Magazine, London, Oct. 20, 1968, pp.26–41.
Portigliotti G: *The Borgias*, (trans. Bernard Miall). George Allen & Unwin, London, 1928.
Praviel A: *Madame de Montespan, empoisonneuse* (Madame Montespan, poisoner). Paris, 1934 (in French).
The Proceedings at Large on the Trial of John Donellan, Esq. for the Wilful Murder (By Poison) of Sir The(odosius) Edward Allesley Boughton. J. Almon & J. Debrett, London, 1781.
Quinn MC: *Doctor Crippen*. Duckworth, London, 1935.
Rabson SM: Doctors delinquent II: the trials of two physicians charged with murder. *JAMA*, 1971;216(1):121–124. (A discussion of the Lamson and Crippen cases.)
Ratzan RM, Ferngren CB: A Greek progymnasma on the physician-poisoner. *J Hist Med Allied Sci* 1993;48(2):157–170.
Raymond E: *A Chorus Ending*. Cassell, London, 1951. (A fictional work based on the Crippen case.)
Raymond E: *We, The Accused: A Novel.* Frederick A. Stokes, New York, NY, 1935. (A novel based on the Crippen case.)
Real-Life Crimes...and How They Were Solved. A magazine series by Eaglemoss Publications Ltd., London, 1993.
#6 - *The Teacup Poisoner*: Graham Young Case
#11 - *A Dose of Poison*: On poisoning investigation
#16 - *The Poisonous Major*: Herbert Armstrong Case
#33 - *Poison Pellet Murder*: Georgi Markov murder
#40 - *Nurse Nancy's Deadly Medicine*: Dorothea Waddingham Case
#66 - *The Paraquat Poisoner*: Susan Barber Case
#67 - *The Poisoned Wine*: Harold Greenwood Case
#86 - *A Poisonous Affair*: Marcus Marymont Case
#93 - *A Victorian Murder*: Adelaide Bartlett Case
#93 - *The Deadly DIY Man*: Cranog James Case
#101 - *Deadly Love Drug*: Arthur Ford Case
#104 - *Death by Prescription*: Paul Vickers Case
#110 - *The Balham Mystery*: Florence Bravo Case
#114 - *An Overdose of Arsenic*: Florence Maybrick Case

Reiterman T, Jacobs J: *Raven: The Untold Story of the Rev. Jim Jones and His People.* Dutton, New York, NY, 1982.

Report of the Trial of Madeleine Smith Before the High Court of Justiciary at Edinburgh...For the Alleged Poisoning of Pierre Emile l'Anglier. T. & T. Clark, Edinburgh, Scotland, 1857.

Reston J: *Our Father Who Art in Hell.* Times Books, New York, NY, 1981. (A discussion of Rev. Jim Jones.)

Reubold W: Poisonings since antiquity. *Gerichtl Med* 1892;43:27.

Robert M: Les empoisonnements criminels au XVIe siecle (Criminal poisoning in 16th century). Storck, *These Med,* Lyon, France, 1903 (in French).

Rosen G: Arrow poisons. *Ciba Symposia;* 1941;3(7):994–1024.

Roughhead W: Poison in the pantry, or Dr. Pritchard revisited, In: *The Murderer's Companion,* The Press of the Readers Club, New York, NY, 1941.

Roughead W: *Malice Domestic.* Green & Son, Edinburgh, Scotland, 1928. (Discussion of the case of Dr. Pritchard, and others.)

Roughead W: *Classic Crimes.* Cassell, London, 1951.

Rowland J: *Poisoner in the Dock: Twelve Studies in Poisoning.* Arco Publications, London, 1960. (Discussions about the following poisoners: Lamson, Pritchard, Charlotte Bryant, Arthur Ford, Adelaide Bartlett, Crippen, Kenneth Barlow, Nurse Waddingham, Mrs. Merrifield, Ethel Major, Louisa Taylor, and Palmer.)

Rowland J: *Murder Revisited: A Study of Two Poisoning Cases.* Longwood, 1961. (Studies of the Major Armstrong, and Harold Greenwood cases.)

Rubinstein N: *Lucrezia Borgia.* Instituto della Enciclopedia Italiana, Rome, Italy, 1971 (in Italian).

Ryan B, Havers M: *The Poisoned Life of Mrs. Maybrick.* Penguin, London, 1989.

Sabatini R: *The Life of Cesare Borgia.* Brentano's, New York, NY, 1923.

Sakula A: "Amadeus" was Mozart poisoned? *History Med,* Jan/Feb 1980;6–9.

Saunders E: *The Mystery of Mary LaFarge.* Pagnerre, Paris, 1840.

Schirokauer A: *Lucretia Borgia* (trans. G. Griffin). Jarrolds, London, 1937.

Schutze J: *Preacher's Girl: The Life and Crimes of Blanche Taylor Moore.* William Morrow & Co., New York, NY, 1993.

Scott H (ed.): *The Concise Encyclopedia of Crime and Criminals.*

Seth R: Petiot: *Victim of Chance.* Hutchinson, London, 1963.

Sheeran G: *The Bradford Poisoning of 1858.* Rayburn Publishing Ltd., Halifax, Canada, 1992.

Smith A: *The Marchioness of Brinvilliers: The Poisoner of the Seventeenth Century. A Romance of Old Paris.* Richard Bentley & Son, London, 1886.

Smith EH: *Famous Poison Mysteries.* The Dial Press, New York, NY, 1927. (Note: published in England as *Famous American Poison Mysteries.* Hurst & Blackett, 1926) (Discussions about the following poisoners: Cordellia Botkin, Carlyle Harris, Dr. Buchanan, Molineux, Dr. Bowers, Mrs. Maybrick, Otto Hoch, Herman Billik, Dr. Crippen, the Wilson Case, Dr. Hyde, Mrs. Schenck, the Twigg-Elosser Case, MacFarland, Louise Vermilya, Annie Monahan, Mrs. Archer-Gilligan, Clarence Richeson, Frederick, Mors, Waite, and Will Orpet.)

Smith S: Poisons and poisoners through the ages. *Med-Legal J* Cambridge, UK, 1952;20(4):153–167.

Somerset A: *Unnatural Murder: Poison at the Court of James I.* Weidenfeld & Nicholson, London, 1997. (A discussion of the murder of Sir Thomas Overbury.)

Sparrow G: *Women Who Murder: Crimes & the Feminine Logic Behind Them.* Abelard-Schuman, New York, NY, 1970.

Sparrow JG: *Vintage Victorian and Edwardian Murder.* Book Club, 1972. (Discussions about the following poisoners: Maybrick, Palmer, the Seddons, and Crippen.)

St. Aubyn G: *Infamous Victorians: Palmer and Lamson—Two Notorious Poisoners.* Constable & Co. Ltd., London, 1971.

Stevenson LG: The Meaning of Poison. *Logan Clendening Lectures on the History and Philosophy of Medicine,* University of Kansas Press, Lawrence, KS, 1959.

Stewart JB: Annals of crime: professional courtesy. *The New Yorker,* Nov. 24, 1997, pp. 90–105. (A discussion of the Michael Swango case).

Stokes H: *Madame de Brinvilliers and Her Times,* 1630–1676.

Stories of Great Crimes & Trials: from American Heritage Magazine, ed. by Oliver Jensen, American Heritage Publishing, New York, NY, 1973.

Swinburne: *Lucretia Borgia.* Golden Cockerel Press, London, 1942.

Swinburne J: *Poisoning by Aconite: Synopsis of the Trial of Hendrickson for the Murder of His Wife.* Philadelphia, PA, 1862.

Symons J: *A Pictorial History of Crime.* Crown Publishers, New York, NY, 1966.

Symons J: *Sweet Adelaide.* Harper & Row, New York, NY, 1980. (Discussion of the Adelaide Bartlett case.)

Tavernier R: *Alors rodait dan l'ombre le docteur Petiot.* Presses de la Cite, Paris, 1974. (in French).

Thompson CJS: *Poison Romance and Poison Mysteries.* The Scientific Press, London, 1899.

Thompson CJS: *Poison Mysteries in History, Romance, and Crime.* J.B. Lippincott, Philadelphia, PA, 1924.

Thompson CJS: *Poisons and Poisoners: With Some Historical Accounts of Some Famous Mysteries in Ancient and Modern Times.* Harold Shaylor, London, 1931.

Thompson CJS: *Poison Mysteries Unsolved: "By Person or Persons Unknown."* Hutchinson & Co., London, 1937.

Thompson CJS: *Magic and Healing: The History and Folklore of Magical Healing Practices from Herb-Lore and Incantations to Rings and Precious Stones.* Bell Publishing, New York, NY, 1989. (Reprint of the 1942 edition.)

Thompson C, Samuel J: *Poisons and Poisoning with Historical Aspects of Some Famous Mysteries.* H. Stysen, London, 1931.

Tichy W: *Poisons: Antidotes & Anecdotes.* Sterling Publishing, New York, NY, 1977.

Thornwald J: *Proof of Poison: How the Great Poisoners Were Brought to Justice —The Story of Toxicology.* Thames & Hudson, London, 1966. (Discussion about the following poisoners: LaFarge, Bodle, Castaing, Bocarme, Pomerais, Lamson, Harris, Seddon, Besnard, Lehmann, and Barlow.)

Thornwald J: The Winding Road of Forensic Toxicology. In: *The Century of the Detective*, Harcourt, Brace & World, New York, NY, 1965, pp. 267–414.

Truc G: *Madame de Montespan*. A. Colin, Paris, 1936. (in French).

Triplett W: *Flowering of the Bamboo*. Woodbine House, Kensington, MD., 1985. (A discussion of the investigation of the Sadamichi Hirasawa case.)

Vance L: *Dr. Crippen*.

Varaut JM: *L'Abominable Dr. Petiot*. Balland, Paris, 1974 (in French).

Villenueve R: *Le Poison et les empoisonneurs celebres* (Poisons and Famous Poisoners). La Palatine, Paris, 1960. (in French).

Vincent A: *A Gallery of Poisoners: Thirteen Classic Case Histories of Murder By Poisoning*. Warner Books, London, 1993. (A discussion of the following poisoners: Seddon, Gburek, Applegate and Creighton, Maybrick, Vaquier, Young, Bartlett, Molineux, Greenwood, Crippen, Cotton, Smith, and Waddingham.)

Voslensky MS: *Das Geheime wird Offenbar. Moskauer Archive erzaehlen* (Secrets Laid Bare. Moscow's Archives Speak Out). (in German).

Wacholz HJ: *Murder by Poisoning (18th & 19th century)*. Mainz, Germany, 1951 (Thesis).

Wacholz LJ: History of poisonings to 19th century. *Przegl Lek (Czech)* 1903; 42:192.

Wagner HJ: Murder by poisoning (18th & 19th Century). *Przegl Lek (Czech)* 1903;42:192.

Wakefield HR: *Landru: The French Bluebeard*. Duckworth, London, 1936.

Waldo FJ, Cantab: Notes on some remarkable British cases of criminal poisoning, No. 1. *Med Brief* 1904;32:4;452-458.

Waldo FJ, Cantab: Notes on some remarkable British cases of criminal poisoning, No. 2, *Med Brief* 1904;32:4;253–259.

Waldo FJ, Cantab: Notes on some remarkable British cases of criminal poisoning, No. 4. *MedBrief* 1904;32:4;936–940.

Walsh C: *The Agra Double Murder*. Ernest Benn, London, 1929.

Watson KD: Highlights in the History of Toxicology, In: *Information Resources in Toxicology*. (Wexler P, ed.), Elsevier, New York, NY, 1982.

Weider B: *Assassination at St. Helena*. Mitchell Press, Vancouver, Canada, 1978.

Weider B, Hapgood D: *The Murder of Napoleon*. Congdon & Lattes, Inc., New York, NY, 1982.

Weider B, Forshufvud S: *Assassination at St. Helena Revisited*. John Wiley, New York, NY, 1995.

Whittington-Egan M: *Khaki Mischief: The Agra Murder Case*. Classic Crime Series, Souvenir, London, 1990.

Wilcox RK: *The Mysterious Deaths at Ann Arbor*. Popular Library, New York, NY, 1977. (A discussion of the acquittal of Leonora Perez and Filipina Narciso case.)

Williams HN: *Madame de Montespan and Louis XIV*, Harper, New York, NY, 1910.

Williams J: *Suddenly at the Priory*. Penguin Books, London, 1989. (Discussion of the Bravo Case.)

Williams P, Wallace D: *Unit 731: Japan's Secret Biological Warfare in World War II*. The Free Press, New York, NY, 1989.

Wittkop-Menardeau G: *Hemlock, ou, Les poisons.* Presses de la Renaissance, Paris, 1988 (in French).

Wood WP: *The Bone Garden: The Sacramento Boardinghouse Murders.* Pocket Books, New York, NY, 1994. (A discussion of the Dorothea Puente case.)

Woodward WH: *Cesare Borgia.* Chapman & Hall, London, 1913.

Young W: *Obsessive Poisoner: The Strange Story of Graham Young.* Robert Hale & Co., London, 1973.

Yriarte C: *Autour des Borgia.* J. Rothschild, Paris, 1891 (in French).

Yriarte C: *Cesare Borgia.* (trans. Wm. Sterling). F. Aldor, London, 1947.

POISONING IN FICTION

Adelson L: The coroner of Elsinore. Some medicolegal reflections on *Hamlet. NEJM* 1960;262(5):229–234.

Agatha Christie, Official Centenary Edition 1890–1990. Harper Paperbacks, Harper-Collins, New York, NY, 1990.

Alexander N: *Poison, Play, and Duel: A Study in Hamlet.* University of NE, Press, Lincoln, NE, 1971.

Bardell EB: Dame Agatha's dispensary. *Pharmacy History* 1984;26(1):13–19.

Bardell EB: Literary reflections of pharmacy. XI: Thallium as "an untraceable poison," *Pharmacy History,* 1988;30:188–190.

Bond RT: *Handbook for Poisoners: A Collection of Great Poison Stories.* Rinehart & Co., New York, NY, 1951.

Borowitz A: *Innocence and Arsenic: Studies in Crime and Literature.* Harper and Row, New York, NY, 1977.

Cooper P: The Devil's foot: an excursion into Holmesian toxicology. *Pharmaceu J* 1966;197:657–658.

Corvasce MV, Paglino JR: *Modus Operandi: A Writer's Guide to How Criminals Work.* The Howdunit Series, Writer's Digest Books, Cincinnati, OH, 1995.

Cromie R, Wilson TS: *The Romance of Poisons: Being Weird Episodes From Life.* Jarrold & Sons, (n.d.).

Done AK: History of poisons in opera. *Mithridata* (newsletter of the Toxicological History Society) 1992;2(2); 3–13.

Fallis G: *Just the Facts Ma'am: A Writer's Guide to Investigators and Investigation Techniques.* The Howdunit Series, Writer's Digest Books, Cincinnati, OH, 1998.

Foster N: Strong Poison - Chemistry in the works of Dorothy L. Sayers, In: *Chemistry and Crime - From Sherlock Holmes to Today's Courtroom,* (Gerber, SM ed.) American Chemical Society, Washington, DC, 1983, pp. 17–29.

Gerald MC: *The Poisonous Pen of Agatha Christie,* University of Texas Press, Austin, Texas, 1993.

Gwilt JR: Brother Cadfael's Herbiary. *Pharmaceut J,* 1992; December 19/26: 807–809.

Gwilt PR, et al.: Dame Agatha's poisonous pharmacopoeia. *Pharmaceut J,* 1978;28, 30:572–573.

Gwilt PR: Poisoning: a dying art. Some observations on the use of poisons in fiction. 1978. (unpublished).

Gwilt PR, et al.: The use of poison in detective fiction. *Clue: A Journal of Detection.* 1981;1:8–17.

Horning J: *The Mystery Lover's Book of Quotations.* The Mysterious Press, New York, NY, 1988.

Huizinga E: Murder through the ear. *Pract Oto-rhino-laryng,* 1971;33:361–365.

Kahn JA: Atropine poisoning in Hawthorne's *The Scarlet Letter. NEJM* 1984;414–416.

Kail AC: Medicine in Shakespeare: The bard and the body, 4. drugs, herbs and poisons. *Med J Australia* Nov. 12, 1983;515–519.

Lundstrom B: Det perfekta mordet Hamlet, Akt I, scen 5 (The perfect murder — Hamlet: Act I, scene 5). *Sydsvenska medicinhistorishka shallskapets jarsskrift* 1977;14:65–77.

Macht DI: Pharmacological appreciation of Shakespeare's *Hamlet:* on instillation of poisons into ear. *Bull Johns Hopkins Hosp* 1918;29:165–170.

Macht DI: A physiological and pharmacological appreciation of *Hamlet* Act 1, Scene 5, Lines 59–73. *Bull Hist of Med* 1949;23:186–194.

Mactire S: *Malicious Intent: A Writer's Guide To How Murderers, Robbers, Rapists and Other Criminals Think.* The Howdunit Series, Writer's Digest Books, Cincinnati, OH, 1995.

Mallory W: *The Mystery Book of Days.* The Mysterious Press, New York, NY, 1990.

Newton HC: *Crime and the Drama, or, Dark Deeds Dramatized.* Stanley Paul & Co., London, 1927. (History of plays based on criminal cases.)

Newton M: *Armed and Dangerous: A Writer's Guide to Weapons.* The Howdunit Series, Writer's Digest Books, Cincinnati, OH, 1990.

Reinert RE: There ARE toadstools in murder mysteries. *MUSHROOM: Journal of Wild Mushrooming.* 1991–92;5–10.

Reinert RE: There ARE toadstools in murder mysteries (Part II). *MUSHROOM: Journal of Wild Mushrooming.* 1994;12(2):9–12.

Reinert RE: More mushrooms in mystery stories. *MUSHROOM—Wild Mushrooming* 1996–97;15(1):5–7.

Silbar H: Michigan's poisoning maniac. *Detective Files* March 1978.

Southward RE, Hollis WG, Thompson DW: Precipitation of a murder: a creative use of strychnine chemistry in Agatha Christie's *The Mysterious Affair at Styles. J Chem Ed* 1992;69(7):536.

Stevens SD, Klarner A: *Deadly Doses: A Writer's Guide to Poisons.* The Howdunit Series, Writer's Digest Books, Cincinnati, OH, 1990.

Tabor E: Plant poisons in Shakespeare. *Econom Botany* 1970;24:81–94.

Thompson CJS: Poisons in fiction, In: *Poison Mysteries in History, Romance, and Crime.* J.B. Lippincott, Philadelphia, PA, 1924, pp. 254–261.

Vourch G: Madame Bovary died of arsenic poisoning. *NEJM* February 14, 1985, p. 446.

Wilson KD: *Cause of Death: A Writer's Guide to Death, Murder and Forensic Medicine.* The Howdunit Series, Writer's Digest Books, Cincinnati, OH, 1992.

Wilson T: Will Shakespeare: Herbalist. *Pharmaceut J* 1992; Dec. 19/26:822–823.

Wingate A: *Scene of the Crime: A Writer's Guide to Crime-Scene Investigations.* The Howdunit Series, Writer's Digest Books, Cincinnati, OH, 1992.

Winn D: *Murder Ink: The Mystery Reader's Companion.* Workman Publishing, New York, NY, 1977.

Winn D: *Murderess Ink: The Better Half of the Mystery.* Workman Publishing, New York, NY, 1979.

FORENSIC POISONING

Aberbathy RJ: Toxicological experiences in the investigation of crime. *Ann Western Med Surg* 1950;4(9):472–473.

Adelson L: Homicidal arsenic poisoning: medicolegal investigation of four cases, Part 1. *Postgrad Med* 1966;39(1):72–86.

Adelson L: Homicidal arsenic poisoning: medicolegal investigation of four cases, Part 2. *Postgrad Med* 1966;39(2):46–60.

Adelson L: Murder by poison, In: *The Pathology of Homicide.* Charles C. Thomas, Springfield, IL, 1974, pp. 725–875.

Adelson L: Homicidal poisoning: a dying modality of lethal violence? *Am J Forensic Med Path* 1987;8(3):245–251.

Ahern D: *How to Commit A Murder.* Ives Washburn, New York, NY, 1930.

Anonymous Poisons and poisoners: old and new. *The Practitioner* 1900;65:171–177; 297–301, 658–663.

Backer RC: Forensic toxicology: a broad overview of general principles, In: *General and Applied Toxicology.* Stockton Press, 1993, pp. 1207–1225.

Bagchi KN: *Poisons and Poisoning: Their History and Romance and Their Detection in Crimes. Kshentamani-Nagendralal Memorial Lectures for 1964,* University of Calcutta, Calcutta, India, 1969.

Barraclough BM: Poisoning cases: suicide or accident. *Br J Psychiat,* 1974, 124, pp. 526–530.

Barrett S: *The Arsenic Milkshake and Other Mysteries Solved By Forensic Science.* Doubleday Canada Ltd, Toronto, Canada, 1994.

Bass G: *Legal Medicine in France 1800–1850.* Juris-Verlag, 1964.

Beck TR: *Elements of Medical Jurisprudence.* Wester & Skinner, Albany, NY, 1823.

Begin E: Legal medicine in France 1971–72, *France Med* 1874;21:218

Bell C: Legal or forensic medicine. *Med-Legal J* 1906/7;24:270.

Bell C: 19th century American medical jurisprudence. *Med-Legal J* 1900/1;18:181.

Bensing RC, Golfarb WB, Schroeder O, et al: Some legal, economic and social aspects of homicide in an urban area. *J Foren Sci,* 1956;1(4):87–89.

Benoit G: De l'empoisonnement criminel (About criminal poisoning). *These Med,* 1888; 407 (in French).

Bernard C: *Lecons sur les effects des substances toxique et medicamenteuse* (Readings on the effects of toxic substances and medications). Paris, France, 1875 (in French).

Bernard C: *Lectures on the Effects of Toxic and Medicinal Substances.* Balliere et Fils, Paris, France, 1857 (in French).

Bili H: A propos de l'empoisonnement criminel (On the topic of criminal poisoning). *These Med,* 1981;339 (in French).

Birkemshaw VJ, et al: Investigation in a case of murder by insulin poisoning. *BMJ* 1958:Aug. 23:463–468.

Bjerre A: *The Psychology of Murder.* Longmans, Green & Co. Ltd., London, 1927.

Black RH: *Directions for the Treatment of Persons Who Have Taken Poison and Those in a State of Apparent Death; Together with the Means of Detecting Poisons and Adulterations in Wine; also, of Distinguishing Real From Apparent Death.*

Nathaniel G. Maxwell, Baltimore, MD, 1819. (Orfila's book translated from the French.)

Blintiff R: *Police Procedural: A Writer's Guide to the Police and How They Work,* Writer's Digest Books, Cincinnati, OH, 1993.

Boar R, Blundell N: *Crooks, Crime and Corruption.* Dorset Press, New York, NY, 1991.

Bodin F, Chenisse CF: *Poisons.* Weidenfield and Nicholson, London, 1970.

Bolitho W: *Murder for Profit.* Harper & Brothers, New York, NY, 1926.

Boos WF: *The Poison Trail.* Hale, Cushman and Flint, Boston, MA, 1939. (Published in as *The Poison Parade.)*

Bouknight R, Alguire P, Lofgren R: A profile of the self-poisoner in Michigan. *Am J Pub Health,* 1985;75:1435–1436.

Bradwell D: Reconstruction of an arsenic poisoning. *J Foren Sci,* 1963;8(2):295–302.

Bresler F: *An Almanac of Murder.* Severn House Publishers, London, 1987.

Brown HM: On poisons. *Ann Med Hist* 1924;6:25–53. (Translation of the 1472 work of Peter Abano.)

Browne DG, Tullett T: *Bernard Spilsbury: Famous Murder Cases of the Great Pathologist.* Panther Books, Granada Publishing Ltd., London, 1982.

Bryson PD: *Comprehensive Review in Toxicology for Emergency Clinicians,* 3rd ed. Taylor & Francis, Washington, DC, 1996.

Burchell HB: Digitalis poisoning: historical and forensic aspects. *J Am Coll Cardiol* 1983;1(2):506–516.

Camps FE, Purchase WB: *Practical Forensic Medicine.* London, 1956.

Caspari-Rosen B (ed.): History of legal medicine. *Ciba Symp* 1950;11(7):1286–1316.

Casper JL: *A Handbook on the Practice of Forensic Medicine based upon Personal Experience...* New Sydenham Soc., London, 1861–65. (four volumes.)

Cavanaugh JB: What have we learnt from Graham Frederick Young? Reflection on the mechanism of thallium neurotoxicity. *Neuropathol Appl Neurobiol,* 1991;17(1):3–9.

Chapman HC: *A Manual of Medical Jurisprudence and Toxicology,* 2nd ed., W.B. Saunders, Philadelphia, PA, 1896.

Charpentier R: Les empoisonneuses. Etude psychologique et medico-legale (Poisonings: Psychologic and Medicolegal Study), *These Med,* 1906;222. (in French).

Chevalier JBA: *Dictionary of Changes and Adulterations of Food, Drug, and Commercial Substances, with an Indication of Ways to Recognize Them.* Bechetheune, Paris, 1850 (in French; 2 vols).

Christison RB: *Treatise on Poisons.* A&C Black, Endinburgh, Scotland, 1829. (2nd ed, 1832; 3rd ed, 1836, 4th ed, 1845.)

Christison RB: *Treatise on Poisons Relation to Jurisprudence.* Barrington, Philadelphia, PA., 1845.

Cina SJ, Raso DS, Conrqadi SE: Suicidal Cyanide ingestion as detailed in *Final Exit. J Foren Sci* 1994;39(6):1568–1570.

Compton JAF: *Military Chemical and Biological Agents: Chemical and Toxicological Properties.* The Telford Press, Caldwell, NJ, 1987.

Cooke MC: *A Treatise on Poisons.* London, 1770.

Cooper C: *Poisoning by Drugs and Chemicals.* Alchemist Press, London, 1974.

Copeman PR, Kamerman PAE: Poisoning by arsenic in South Africa. *South African Med J* 1940;14:473.

Copeman P, Bodenstein J: An investigation of cases of arsenical poisoning. *J Foren Med* 1955;2(4):196–216.

Cordess C: Criminal poisoning and the psychopathology of the poisoner. *J Foren Psychiatr* 1990;1(2):213–226.

Corvasce MV, Paglino JR: *Murder One: A Writer's Guide to Homicide.* Writer's Digest Books, Cincinnati, OH, 1997.

Crimes Involving Poison. Department of the Army Technical Bulletin TB PMG 21, Department of the Army, Washington, DC, 1967.

Crow WE: Criminal poisoning in Hong Kong. Lecture before Odd Volumes in Hong Kong. *Rev Pharm Rev* 14:164.

Cummings J: *Bibliography of Crime.* Patterson Smith, Montclair, NJ, 1970.

Cumston CG: XVI poisoning cases aspects medicolegal. *Med-Legal J* 1905, 23:172.

Cuthbert TM: A portfolio of murders. *Br J Psychiatry* 1970;116:1–10.

Dearden H: *The Mind of the Murderer.* Sears Publishing Co. Inc., New York, NY, 1930. (Discussion of the following poisoners: Armstrong, Cream, Crippen, LaFarge, Mercier, Seddon, Troppmann, and Zwanziger.)

Deaths by poison: Return of Inquests. Government Publication, UK 1839;(585); xxxviii; 409.

Dewachter P: A propos d'une femme inculpee d'empoisonnement, Memoire diplome d'universite de criminologie (On the topic of an indicted female. *Dissertation certificate of the University of Criminology*). Nancy, France 1987, p. 40 (in French).

Dewachter P, Diligent MB, Hennequin JP, et al: A propos d'une femme empoisonneuse-reflexions psychologiques et criminologiques (On the subject of a female poisoner. Psychological and criminological considerations). *J Med Legal Droit Med* 1989;34(4):343–349 (in French).

Dietz PE: Dangerous information: product tampering and poisoning advice in revenge and murder manuals. *J Foren Sci* 1988;33(5):1206–1217.

Dine M, McGovern M: Intentional poisoning of children: an overlooked category of child abuse. Report of 7 cases and review of the literature. *Pediatrics* 1982;70:32–35.

D'Orban PT, O'Connor A: Women who kill their parents. *Brit J Psychiatr* 1989; 154:27–33.

Doremus RO: Duties of experts and others in poison cases. *Criminal Law Magazine,* Jersey City, NJ, 1880.

Douglas JE, Burgess AW, Burgess AG, et al: *Crime Classification Manual—A Standard System for Investigating and Classifying Violent Crimes.* Lexington Books, New York, NY, 1992.

Douglas JE, Olshaker M: *Mind Hunter: Inside the FBI's Elite Serial Crime Unit.* Scribner, New York, NY, 1995. (Discussion of the, 1982 Tylenol tampering incident, pp. 318–324.)

Douglas JE, Olshaker M: *Journey into Darkness: Follow the FBI's Premier Investigative Profiler as He Penetrates the Minds and Motives of the Most Terrifying Serial Criminals.* Scribner, New York, NY, 1997.

Draper FW: *A Textbook of Legal Medicine.* W.B. Saunders, Philadelphia, PA, 1905.

Duncklemeyer E: Uber seltene arten krimineller giftbeibringun (Rare forms of criminal administration of poisons—I). *Archiv fur Kriminol* 1986;178(1–2):35–43 (in German).

Duncklemeyer E: Uber seltene arten krimineller giftbeibringun (Rare forms of criminal administration of poisons—II), *Archiv fur Kriminol* 1986;178(3–4):95–102 (in German).

Dundee JW: Mysterious deaths at Ann Arbor. *Anesthesia* 1978;33:752–753.

Eckert WG: Mass deaths by gas or chemical poisoning: A historical perspective. *Am J Forensic Med Pathol* 1991;12(2):119–125.

Ellenhorn MJ: *Ellenhorn's Medical Toxicology: Diagnosis and Treatment of Human Poisoning.* (2nd Ed.). Williams & Wilkins, Baltimore, MD, 1996.

Embry JH, Walls HC: Serial arsenic poisoning: two Alabama cases. *Alabama Med* 1990;59(10):24–28.

Emerson RL: *Legal Medicine and Toxicology.* Appleton & Co., New York, NY, 1909.

Epivatianos P, Tsoukali-Papadopoulous E: Un case rare d'intoxication criminelle de trois enfants par leur mere au cours d'une periode de 10 mois (A singular case of criminal drug intoxication of three children by their mother during a period of ten months). *Revue Internationale de Criminologie et de Police Technique* 1990;43(1):91–93 (in French).

Ewell MD: *A Manual of Medical Jurisprudence, General Toxicology.* Little, Brown & Co., Boston, MA, 1887.

Fallis G: *Just The Facts Ma'am: A Writer's Guide to Investigators and Investigation Techniques.* Writer's Digest Books, Cincinnati, OH, 1998.

Farr S: Elements of Medical Jurisprudence. London, 1787. (2nd ed., 1814).

Farrell M: *Poisons and Poisoners: An Encyclopedia of Homicidal Poisonings.* Robert Hale, London, 1992.

Faselius JF: *Elementa Medicinae Forensis.* Geneva, Switzerland, 1767.

Fein RA, Vossekuil B, Holden GA: Threat assessment: an approach to prevent targeted violence. *Research in Action,* Office of Justice Programs, National Institute of Justice, September 1995, pp. 1–7.

Ferner RE: *Forensic Pharmacology: Medicines, Mayhem, and Malpractice.* Oxford University Press, New York, NY, 1996.

Fester U: *Silent Death.* Loompanics Unlimited, Port Townsend, WA, 1989. (2nd ed., revised and expanded, 1997.) (An underground press book on how to kill with poisons.)

Fingerhut LA, Cox CS: Poisoning mortality: 1985–1995. *Public Health Reports,* 1998;111:219–233.

Fisher BAJ: *Techniques of Crime Scene Investigation,* 5th ed. CRC Press, Boca Raton, FL, 1993.

Furneux R: *The Medical Murderer.* Abelard-Schuman, New York, NY, 1966.

Gradwohl RHB: *Leg Med.* St. Louis, Missouri, 1953.

Geberth VJ: *Practical Homicide Investigation: Tactics, Procedures, and Forensic Techniques,* 2nd ed. Elsevier, New York, NY, 1990.

Gee DJ: Cyanides in murder, suicide, and accident, In: *Clinical and Experimental Toxicology of Cyanides,* Ballantyne, B; Marrs, TC, eds. PSG Publishing Littleton, MA, 1987, pp. 209–216.

Glaister J, Rentoul E: *Medical Jurisprudence and Toxicology.* 12th ed. Livingstone, Edinburgh, Scotland, 1966.

Glaser H: *Poison: the History, Constitution, Uses and Abuses of Poisonous Substances.* Hutchinson, London, 1937.

Goldfrank LR, Flomenbaum NE, Lewin NA et al.: *Goldfrank's Toxicologic Emergencies,* 6th ed. Appleton and Lange, Stamford, CT, 1998.

Gonzales TA, Vance BM, Helpern M et al.: *Legal Medicine, Pathology and Toxicology,* 2nd ed. New York, NY, 1954.

Gordon I, Turner R, Price TW: *Medical Jurisprudence,* 3rd ed. Edinburgh, Scotland, 1953.

Goulding R: Poisoning as a fine art. *Med-Legal J* 1978;46:6–17.

Goulding R: Poisoning as a social phenomenon. *J Royal Coll Phys Lond* 1987;21:282–286.

Guillen T: *Toxic Love.* Dell Publishing, New York, NY, 1995. (A discussion of the Steven Ray Harper case.)

Guttmacher MS: *The Mind of the Murderer.* Farrar Straus, New York, NY, 1960.

Haddad LM, Shannon MW, Winchester JF: *Clinical Managing of Poisoning and Drug Overdose,* 3rd ed. W.B. Saunders Co., Philadelphia, PA, 1998.

Haines WS: *Legal Medicine and Toxicology.* W.B. Saunders, Philadelphia, PA. vol. 1, 1903; vol. 2, 1904; 2nd ed.; vol. 2, 1923.

Hanzlick R, Combs D, Parrish RG, et al: Death investigation in the United States, 1990: a survey of statutes, systems, and educational requirements. *J Foren Sci* 1993;38(3):628–632.

Harber D: *Assorted Nasties.* Desert Publications, Eldorado, AR, 1993. (The "ultimate handbook on poisons and application devices." An underground press book on how to kill with poisons.)

Harry B: Criminals' explanations of their criminal behavior, Part I: the contribution of criminologic variables. *J Foren Sci* 1992;37(5):1327–1333.

Harry B: Criminals' explanations of their criminal behavior, Part II: a possible role for psychopathy. *J Foren Sci* 1992;37(5):1334–1340.

Harris R, Paxman J: *A Higher Form of Killing: The Secret Story of Chemical and Biological Warfare.* Hill and Wang, New York, NY, 1982.

Harvard JDJ: *The Detection of Secret Homicide: A Study of the Medico-legal System of Investigation of Sudden and Unexplained Deaths.* Macmillan & Co. London, 1960.

Hemming WD: *Forensic Medicine and Toxicology.* Putnam, New York, NY, 1889.

Herold J: *A Manual of Legal Medicine.* J.B. Lippincott, Philadelphia, PA, 1898.

Hine CH, Hall FB, Turkel HW: Forensic toxicology and the practicing physician. *Clin Tox* 1968;1(1):71–80.

Holland J: *A Textbook of Medical Chemistry and Toxicology.* Philadelphia, PA, 1905.

Howells K: The meaning of poisoning to a person diagnosed as a psychopath. *Med Sci Law* 1978;18(3):179–184.

Hutchkinson M: *The Poisoner's Handbook.* Loompanics Unlimited, Port Townsend, WA, 1988. (an underground press book on how to kill with poisons.)

Hyde M, et al.: *Crimes and Punishment,* 8 vols. Marshall Cavendish Corp., Freeport, NY, 1986.

Jesse FT: *Murder and its Motives,* George G. Harrap & Co., London, 1924.

Kelleher MD, Kelleher CL: *Murder Most Rare: The Female Serial Killer.* Praeger Publishers, Westport, CT, 1998.
Kerr DJA: *Forensic Medicine,* 5th ed. A&C Black, London, 1954.
Kirwin BR: *The Mad, the Bad, and the Innocent: The Criminal Mind on Trial—Tales of a Forensic Psychologist.* Little Brown & Co., New York, NY, 1997.
Knight B: Ricin: a potent homicidal poison. Medicolegal, *BMJ* 1979;350–351.
Kobert R: *Practical Toxicology for Physicians and Students,* Friedburg, LH, WR Jenkins, eds. 1897. New York, NY, (1st American edition.)
Kroll P, Silk K, Chamberlain K, et al.: Denying the incredible: unexplained deaths in a veterans administration hospital. *Am J Psychiatr,* 1977;134(12):1376–1380.
Kunkel AK: *Handbuch der Toxikologie* (Handbook of Toxicology). G. Fisher, Jena, 1899. (in German).
Kurland M: *How To Solve A Murder: The Forensic Handbook.* Macmillan, New York, NY, 1995.
Kurland M: *How To Try A Murder: The Handbook for Armchair Lawyers.* Macmillan, New York, NY, 1997.
Leipmann H: *Poison in the Air.* J.B. Lippincott, London, 1937. (A discussion of the history and elements of chemical warfare.)
Logan B: Product tampering crime: a review. *J Foren Sci* 1993;38(4):918–927.
Logan B, Howard J, Kiesel EL: Poisonings associated with cyanide in over the counter cold medication in Washington state, 1991. *J Foren Sci* 1993;38(2):472–476.
Lucas A: *Forensic Chemistry and Scientific Criminal Investigation.* 2nd ed. London, 1931.
Luff AP: *Text-Book of Forensic Medicine and Toxicology.* Longmans, Green, London, 1895.
Lynch GR: Poisons and poisoning. *Med-Legal Rev* 1942, 193–202.
Male GE: *Epitome of Judicial and Forensic Medicine.* London, 1816.
Mangin A: *Le Poisons* (Poisons). Alfred Mame Et Fils, Tours, France, 1869. (in French).
Mann JD: *Forensic Medicine and Toxicology.* P. Blackinston's Sons, Philadelphia, PA, 1893. (4th ed, 1908.)
Marriner B: *On Death's Bloody Trail: Murder and the Art of Forensic Science.* St. Martin's Press, New York, NY, 1993.
Massey EW, Wold D, Heyman A: Arsenic: homicidal intoxication. *Southern Med J* 1984;77(7):848–851.
Mathys R: Neuf observations d'empoisonnement criminel par le Thallium (Nine observations on criminal poisoning by Thallium). *Annales de Medicine Legale et de Criminologie* 1955;35:237–275 (in French).
Matthys R, Thomas F: Criminal Thallium poisoning. *J Foren Med* 1958;5:111–121.
Mawson D: Delusions of poisoning. *Med Sci Law* 1985;25(4):279–187.
McCormack J, McKinney W: Thallium poisoning in group assassination attempt. *Postgrad Med* 1983;74(6):239–244.
McLaughlin T: *The Coward's Weapon.* Robert Hale Ltd., London, 1980.
McNally WD: *Medical Jurisprudence and Toxicology.* W.B. Saunders, Philadelphia, PA, 1939.

Mead R: *A Mechanical Account of Poisons in Several Essays: I "Of the Viper", II "Of the Tarantula and the Mad Dog", III "Of Poisonous Minerals and Plants, IV "Of Opium", and V "On Venomous Exhalations from the Earth, Poisonous Airs, and Waters,"* printed by J.R. for Ralph South, London, 1702. (3rd ed. 1745, 4th ed. 1747) (Note: this is the first book written in English on the subject of poisons.)

Meadow R: Poisoning. *BMJ* 1989;298:1445–1446.

Megargee EI: *Classifying Criminal Offenders*. Sage, Beverly Hills, CA, 1979.

Meggs WJ, Hoffman RS, Shih RD et al.: Thallium poisoning from maliciously contaminated food. *Clin Toxicol* 1994; 32(6):723–730.

Melow JR, McEllistrem JE: Bombing and psychopathy: an investigative review. *J Foren Sci* 1998;43(3):556–562.

Melton HK: *The Ultimate Spy Book.* DK Publishing Co., New York, NY, 1996. (Includes discussions of some assassination weapons utilizing poisons, and victims.)

Modi JP: *Modi's Textbook of Medical Jurisprudence and Toxicology,* 19th ed. NM Tripathi, Bombay, India, 1975.

Moffat AC: Forensic pharmacognosy: poisoning with plants. *J Foren Sci Soc* 1980;20(2):103–109.

Moller D: To catch a blackmailer. *Reader's Digest,* April 1992, pp. 68–228.

Moore K, Reed D: *Deadly Medicine.*

Murphy D: The self-poisoner: a profile. *Public Health (England)* 1982;96(3):148–154.

Nash JR: *Crime Chronology: A Worldwide Record. 1900–1983,* Facts on File Publications, New York, NY, 1984.

Neustatter WL: *The Mind of the Murderer*. Philosophical Library, New York, NY, 1957.

Nordby JJ: Can we believe what we see, if we see what we believe? Expert disagreement. *J Foren Sci* 1992;37(4):1115–1124.

O'Hara CE: Homicide, In: *Fundamentals of Criminal Investigation*. Charles C. Thomas Publishers, Springfield, IL, 1956, pp. 373–476.

Oliver JS, Smith H, Watson AA: Poisoning by strychnine. *Med Sci Law* 1979;19(2):134–137.

Orfila MJB: *Traite des Poisons*. Chez Crochard, Paris, France, 1814 (2 vol) (Note: this is the first book written on General Toxicology) (in French).

Orfila MJB: *Appendix to the General System of Toxicology or, A Treatise on Mineral, Vegetable, and Animal Poisons...to which are added twenty-two coloured engravings of poisonous plants, fungi, insects, etc.,* (trans. by J.A. Waller). E. Cox, London, 1821. (An appendix for the original 1814 edition *Traite des Poisons.*)

Orfila MJB: *Recherches Medico-Legales et Therapeutiqies sur l'Empoisonnement par l'Acide Arsenieux...Recuillies et Redigees par le Docteur Beaufort.* Paris, France, 1842. (in French).

Orfila MP: *A Practical Treatise on Poisons and Asphyxies, adapted to general use, (translated from the French by JG Stevenson).* Hilliard, Gray, Little, and Wilkins; Boston, MA, 1826.

Page DW: *Body Trauma: A Writer's Guide to Wounds and Injuries.* Writer's Digest Books, Cincinnati, OH, 1996.

Palmer S: *The Psychology of Murder.* Thomas Y. Crowell Company, New York, NY, 1962.

Parker J: *The Killing Factory: The Top Secret World of Germ and Chemical Warfare.* Smith Gryphon, England.

Paton GA: Development of forensic toxicology. *Proc Med Legal Soc Victoria* 1941;4:241.

Peterson F, Haines WS: *A Textbook of Legal Medicine and Toxicology.* W.B. Saunders, Philadelphia, PA: (vol 1, 1903; vol 2, 1904).

Petursson H, Gudjonnson GH: Psychiatric aspects of homicide. *Acta Psychiat Scand.* 1981;64:363–372.

Picton B: *Murder, Suicide, or Accident.* St. Martin's Press, New York, NY, 1971.

Poklis A, Saady JJ: Arsenic poisoning: acute or chronic? Suicide or murder? *Am J Foren Med Pathol* 1990;11(3):226–232.

Pollak O: *The Criminality of Women.* Greenwood Press, Westport, CT, 1978.

Polson CJ: *Essentials of Forensic Medicine.* London, 1955.

Polson CJ, Green MA, Lee MR: *Clinical Toxicology,* 3rd ed. J.B. Lippincott, Philadelphia, PA, 1983.

Popkess A: Morphia the slayer. *Police J* 1952;25:248–257.

Prestwich R: *Prestwich's Dissertation on Mineral, Animal, and Vegetable Poisons.* London, 1775.

Price W, *A Popular Treatise on the Remedies to be Employed in Cases of Poisoning and Apparent Death, Including the Means of Detecting Poisons, of Distinguishing Real from Apparent Death and of Ascertaining the Adulteration of Wines.* 1818.

Prick JJG, Smitt WGS, Muller L: *Thallium Poisoning.* Elsevier, Amsterdam, 1955.

Quatrehomme G, Ricq O, Lapalus P, et al: Acute arsenic intoxication: forensic and toxicologic aspects (an observation). *J Foren Sci* 1992;37(4):1163–1171.

Reese JJ: *Textbook of Medical Jurisprudence and Toxicology.* P. Blakiston's Sons & Co., Philadelphia, PA, 1884 (3rd ed., 1891).

Rendle-Short J: Non-accidental barbiturate poisoning of children. *Lancet* 1978;2:1212.

Ressler RK, Shachtman T: *Whoever Fights Monsters.* St. Martin's Press, New York, NY, 1992.

Ressler RK, Shachtman T: *I Have Lived in the Monster.* St. Martin's Press, New York, NY, 1997.

Riley CM: *Toxicology: The Nature, Effects and Detection of Poisons, with the Diagnosis and Treatment of Poisoning.* St. Louis Medical Book Publishing, St. Louis, MO, 1902.

Roche LG: Death simulating natural causes. *Med-Legal Criminological Rev* 1942;10:69.

Rogers D, Tripp J, Bentovin A, et al.: Non-accidental poisoning: an extended syndrome of child abuse. *BMJ* 1976;1:793–796.

Rose PB: *Hand-book of Toxicology.* Courier Stream Printing House, Ann Arbor, MI, 1880.

Rosenberg ML, Davidson LE, Smith JC et al.: Operational criteria for the determination of suicide. *J Foren Sci* 1988;33(6):1445–1456.

Roth M: *The Writer's Complete CRIME Reference Book.* Writer's Digest Books, Cincinnati, OH, 1990.

Roueche B: *The Medical Detectives.* Times Books, New York, NY, 1981.

Roueche B: *The Medical Detectives, vol II.* E.P. Dutton, Inc., New York, NY, 1984.

Ruta D, Haider S: Attempted murder by Selenium poisoning. *BMJ* 1989;299:316–317.

Ryan M: *Manual of Medical Jurisprudence.* London, 1832.

Saulsbury F, Chobanian M, Wilson W: Child abuse: parental hydrocarbon administration. *Pediatrics* 1984;73(5):719–722.

Semple CEA: *Essentials of Legal Medicine, Toxicology, and Hygiene.* Philadelphia, PA, 1892.

Shew ES: *A Companion to Murder: A Dictionary of Death by Poison, 1900–1950.* Alfred A. Knopf, New York, NY, 1961.

Shew ES: *A Second Companion to Murder: A Dictionary of Death by Knife,*1900–1950, Alfred A. Knopf, New York, NY, 1962.

Siegel H, Reiders F, Holmstedt B: The medical and scientific evidence in alleged tubocurarine poisonings. A review of the so-called Dr. X case. *Foren Sci Intl* 1985;29:29–76.

Simon RI: Murder masquerading as suicide: postmortem assessment of suicide risk factors at the time of death. *J Forensic Sci* 1998;43(6):1119–1123.

Simpson K: Murder by arsenic. *Police J* 1949;22:263–268.

Simpson K: Carbon monoxide poisoning: medico-legal problems. *J Foren Med* 1955;2(1):5–13.

Simpson K: *Forensic Medicine,* 3rd ed., London, 1958.

Simpson K (ed.): *Modern Trends in Forensic Medicine.* London, 1953.

Smith H: The psychology of the poisoner, In: *Famous Poison Trials.* W. Collins Sons & Co. Ltd., London, 1923, pp. 1–10.

Smith S, Fiddes FS: *Forensic Medicine.* Churchill, London, 1955.

Smyth F: *Cause of Death: A History of Forensic Science.* Pan Books, London, 1980.

Sparrow G: *Women Who Murder: Crimes and the Feminine Logic Behind Them.* Abelard-Schuman Ltd., New York, NY, 1970.

Starrs JE: Misery loves...death! Nurses who kill: a fatal and virulent toxin. *Scientific Sleuthing Review—Forensic Science in Law Enforcement* 1992;16(3):1–5.

Stehlin IB: FDA's forensic center: speedy, sophisticated sleuthing. *FDA Consumer,* July-August 1995;5–9.

Stephenson J: *Medical Zoology, and Mineralology; or Illustrations and Descriptions of the Animals and Minerals Employed in Medicine, and of the Preparations Derived from Them; including also an Account of Animal and Mineral Poisons.* London, 1838.

Szymusik A: Studies on the psychopathology of murderers. *Polish Med J* 1972;11(3):752–757.

Tanner TH: *Memoranda on Poisons.* Blakison, Philadelphia, PA, 1901.

Tardieu A: *Etude medico-legale et clinique sur l'Empoisonnement...*(Med-legal and clinical studies on poisons). J.B. Balliere, Paris,1975 (in French).

Tardieu A: *L'Empoisonement* (Poisons) 2nd ed. Bailliere et fils, Paris, 1875 (in French).

Taylor AS: *On Poisons in Relation to Medical Jurisprudence and Medicine.* Lea & Blanchard, Philadelphia, PA, 1848.

Taylor AS: *On poisoning by strychnine with comments on the medical evidence given at the trial of William Palmer for the murder of John Parsons Cook.* Longman, Brown, Green, Longmans & Ruberts, London, 1856. (Reprinted from the Guy's Hospital Report for October 1856, with additional notes and cases.)

Taylor AS: *A Treatise on Poisons in Relation to Medical Jurisprudence and Medicine,* 3rd ed. Henry C. Lea, Philadelphia, PA, 1875.

Teare GD: A case of homicidal poisoning. *Police J* 1954;27:194–199.

Teare D, Brown S: Poisoning by paraquat. *Med-Legal J* 1976;44(2)33–47.

The Guyana tragedy: an international forensic problem. *Foren Sci Int* 1979;13(2):167–174.

Thompson CJS: The psychology of the criminal poisoner, In: *Poison Mysteries Unsolved—"By Person or Persons Unknown,"* Hutchinson and Co., London, 1937, pp. 15–20.

Thorwald J: *The Century of the Detective.* Harcourt Brace and World, New York, NY, 1965.

Thorwald J: *Crime and Science: The New Frontier in Criminology.* Harcourt Brace and World, New York, NY, 1967.

Toxic techniques, Legal Medicine, *MD* October 1959, pp. 139–143.

Turner WW (ed.): *Drugs and Poisons.* Police Evidence Library, Aqueduct Books, 1965.

Vandome N: *Crimes and Criminals.* Chamber's Encyclopedic Guides, W & R Chambers Ltd., New York, NY, 1992.

Van Hecke V: A case of murder by parathion (E 605) which nearly escaped detection. *Med Sci and Law* 1964;4:197–199.

Vibert C: *Precis de toxicologie clinique et medico-legale...* J.B. Balliere, Paris, 1900 (in French).

Weiler G: Ein ungewohnlicher cyanid-mord (An unusual cyanide murder). *Archiv fur Kriminologie* 1983;16–20 (in German).

Westeveer AE, Trestrail JH, Pinizzotto J: Homicidal poisonings in the United States: An analysis of the Uniform Crime Reports from 1980 through 1989. *Am J Foren Med Pathol* 1996;17(4)282–288.

Wigmore JH: Circumstantial evidence in poisoning cases. *Clinics (Philadelphia)* 1943;1(6):1,507–1,519.

Wilber CG: *Forensic Toxicology for the Law Enforcement Officer.* Charles C. Thomas, Springfield, IL, 1980.

Wilcox RH: *The Mysterious Deaths at Ann Arbor.* Popular Library, New York, NY, 1977.

Willcox W: Toxicology with reference to its criminal aspects. *West London Med J* 1938;43:133–153.

Wilson C, Pitman P: *Encyclopedia of Murder.* London, 1961.

Wilson C, Seaman C: *The Encyclopedia of Modern Murder.* Arlington House, New York, NY, 1988.

Wilson C: *The Mammoth Book of True Crime,* vols. 1 and 2. Carrol & Graf Publishers, Inc., New York, NY, 1990.

Witthaus RA: *Medical Jurisprudence Forensic Medicine and Toxicology.* William Wood, New York, NY (four vols.: vol. 1 and 2, 1894; vols. 3 and 4, 1896.)

Witthaus RA: *Manual of Toxicology.* Bailliere Tindall and Cox, London, 1911.

Wood HC: *A Treatise on Therapeutics: Comprising Materia Medica and Toxicology,* 3rd ed. J.B. Lippincott, Philadelphia, PA, 1880.

Woodman WB, Tidy CM: *Forensic Medicine and Toxicology.* Philadelphia, PA, 1882.

Wormley TG: *Micro-Chemistry of Poisons...* William Wood, New York, NY, 1869. (Note: this is the first book printed in the US devoted entirely to the subject of toxicology.)

Young DB, McCormick GM: There's death in the cup, so beware! *Am J Foren Med Pathol* 1995;16(3):223–228.

ANALYTIC TOXICOLOGY

Autenrieth W, Warren WH: *The Detection of Poisons and Strong Drugs. Including the Quantitative Estimation of Medicinal Principles in Certain Crude Materials.* P. Blakiston's Son & Co., Philadelphia, PA, 1905.

Baselt RC, Cravey RH: *Disposition of Toxic Drugs and Chemicals in Man,* 3rd ed. Year Book Medical Publishers, Chicago, IL, 1989.

Blyth AW: *Poisons and Their Effects and Detection: A Manual for the Use of Analytical Chemists and Experts.* Charles Griffin, London, 1884. (2 vols.; U.S. edition, published by William Wood, New York, NY, 1885.)

Campbell WA: Some landmarks in the history of arsenic testing. *Chemistry Britain* 1965;1:198–202.

Cavendish M: *Science Against Crime.*

Chiavarelli S: Toxicologic chemistry, historic and contemporary. *Ann Ist Sup San* 1968;4:445.

Clarke EGC: *Isolation and Identification of Drugs in Pharmaceuticals, Body Fluids, and Post–Mortem Material.* The Pharmaceutical Press, London, 1969.

Coe JI: Postmortem chemistry: practical considerations and a review of the literature. *J Foren Sci* 1974,19(1):13–32.

Collin E: *Traite de toxicologie vegetale. Application du microscope a la recherche des poisons vegetaux...* O. Dolin, Paris, 1907 (in French).

Curry AS: *Poison Detection in Human Organs.* Charles C. Thomas, Springfield, IL, 1976.

Druid H, Holmgren P: A compilation of fatal and control concentrations of drugs in postmortem femoral blood. *J Foren Sci* 1997;42(1):79–87.

Gerber SM: *Chemistry and Crime: From Sherlock Holmes to Today's Courtroom.* American Chemical Society, Washington, DC, 1983.

Gerber SM, Saferstein R: *More Chemistry and Crime: From Marsh Arsenic Test to DNA Profile.* American Chemical Society, Washington, DC, 1997.

Hilberg T, Rogde S, Morland J: Postmortem drug distribution: human cases related to results in experimental animals. *J Foren Sci* 1999;44(1):3–9.

Imwinkelried EJ: Forensic science: toxicological procedures to identify poisons. *CR Law Bull* 1994;30:172–179.

Itallie I: Fixation of time and administration in cases of chronic arsenic poisoning. *Anal,* 1937;62:401.

Jones GR, Pounder DJ: Site dependence of drug concentrations in postmortem blood: A case study. *J Anal Toxicol* 1987;11.

LeBeau M, Andollo W, Hearn LE, et al: Recommendation for toxicological investigations of drug-facilitated sexual assaults. *J Foren Sci* 1999;44(1):227–230.

Loga BK, Smirnow D: Postmortem distribution and redistribution of morphine in man. *J Foren Sci* 1996;41(2):37–46.

Langford AM, Pounder DJ: Possible markers for postmortem drug redistribution. *J Foren Sci* 1997;42(1):88–92.

Mitchell CA: *Forensic Chemistry in the Criminal Courts.* The Institute of Chemistry, London, 1938.

Moriya F, Hashimoto Y: Redistribution of basic drugs into cardiac blood from surrounding tissues during early-stages postmortem. *J Foren Sci* 1999,44(1):10–16.

Moyer TP: Heavy metals: the forgotten toxins. *Therapeut Drug Monitoring Clin Toxicol* 199611(3):1–5.

Niyogi SK: Historic development of forensic toxicology in America up to 1978. *Am J Foren Med Pathol* 1980;1(3):249–264. (204 references.)

Niyogi SK: Historical overview of forensic toxicology, In: *Introduction to Forensic Toxicology.* Cravey RH, Baselt RC, eds. Biomedical Publications, Davis, CA, 1981, pp. 7–24.

Pirl JN, Townsend GF, Valaitis AK (et al.): Death by arsenic: a comparative evaluation of exhumed body tissues in the presence of external contamination. *J Anal Toxicol* 1983;7(5):216–219.

Pounder DJ: The nightmare of postmortem drug changes, In: *Legal Medicine 1993.* Butterworth Legal Publishers, 1993, pp. 163–191.

Pounder DJ, Jones GR: Post-mortem drug distribution: a toxicological nightmare. *Foren Sci Int* 1990;45:253–263.

Pounder DJ, Owen V, Quigley C: Postmortem changes in blood amitriptyline concentration. *Am J Foren Med Pathol* 1994;15(3):224–230.

Repetto RM, Repetto M: Habitual, toxic, and lethal concentrations of 103 drugs of abuse in humans. *Clin Toxicol* 1997;35(1):1–9.

Repetto RM, Repetto M: Therapeutic, toxic, and lethal concentrations in human fluids of 90 drugs affecting the cardiovascular and hematopoietic systems. *Clin Toxicol* 1997;35(4):345–351.

Repetto MR, Repetto M: Therapeutic, toxic, and lethal concentrations of 73 drugs affecting respiratory system in human fluids. *Clin Toxicol* 1998;36(4):287–293.

Reyes LL, Santos JG: Importance of information in forensic toxicology. *Am J Foren Med Pathol* 1992;13(1):33–36.

Risser D, Bonsch A, Schneider B: Should coroners be able to recognize unintentional Carbon monoxide deaths immediately at the death scene? *J Foren Sci* 1995;40(4):596–598.

Rule G, McLaughlin LG, Henion J: A quest for oleandrin in decayed human tissue. *Anal Chem* 1993;65(19):857A.

Walker JT: Scientific evidence in poisoning cases. *Clinics* 1943;1(6):1520–1535.

Wilson B: Traces of poison. *Chem Britain,* May 1993;405–406.

Zeldenrust J, Boer D: Fatal phosphorus poisoning elucidated by exhumation three and a half years after burial. *Med Sci & Law* 1964;4:120–121.

INDEX

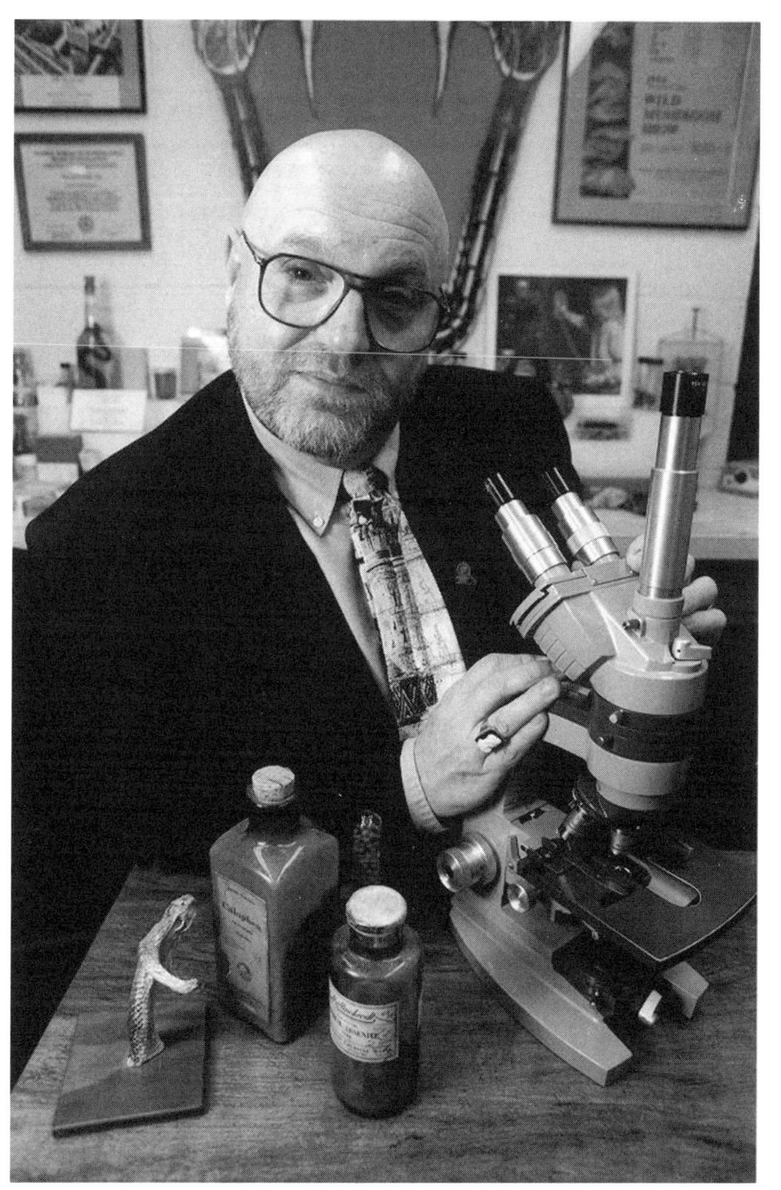

About the Author

John Harris Trestrail, III, RPh, FAACT, DABAT
Toxicologist

Dr. Trestrail graduated with honors, obtaining a B.S. degree in Pharmacy, from Ferris State University, Big Rapids, Michigan, in 1967, where he was initiated into Rho Chi (Pharmaceutical Honors Society). From 1967 to 1968 he attended graduate school, majoring in natural product chemistry at the College of Pharmacy, The Ohio State University, Columbus, Ohio. Dr. Trestrail's public service experience was with the United States Peace Corps, from 1968 to 1970, where he taught chemistry at the University of the Philippines College of Agriculture, in the Republic of the Philippines. He is a practicing boarded toxicologist, and is a visiting instructor at the FBI National Academy in Quantico, Virginia. Since 1976, he has served as the Managing Director of one of the nation's certified regional poison centers.

He has been honored as a Fellow by the American Academy of Clinical Toxicology, and is a Diplomate, by examination, of the American Board of Applied Toxicology. Dr. Trestrail founded the Center for the Study of Criminal Poisoning, as well as the Toxicological History Society, and has been featured in several episodes of *"The New Detectives,"* on the Discovery Channel. He is a participant in the International Program on Clinical Safety of the World Health Organization (WHO). Dr. Trestrail has also served in many criminal poisoning investigations as an expert consultant to law enforcement and attorneys. Since 1990, Dr. Trestrail's seminars on *"Murder by Poison!"* and *"Poisoners Throughout History"* have been received with wide acclaim by audiences throughout the United States, Canada, and Europe.

John and Mary Trestrail have been married since 1971, and are the parents of two now adult children, John and Amanda.

Dr. Trestrail is a member of the following professional organizations: The American Academy of Clinical Toxicology (AACT), The American Association of Poison Control Centers (AAPCC), The International Association of Forensic Toxicologists (TIAFT), The International Homicide Investigators Association (IHIA), The International Society on Toxinology (IST), The North American Mycological Association (NAMA), The Society of Forensic Toxicologists (SOFT), and The Toxicological History Society (THiS).